Disorders of the Chest Wall

Editor

HENNING A. GAISSERT

THORACIC SURGERY CLINICS

www.thoracic.theclinics.com

Consulting Editor
M. BLAIR MARSHALL

May 2017 • Volume 27 • Number 2

ELSEVIER

1600 John F. Kennedy Boulevard • Suite 1800 • Philadelphia, Pennsylvania, 19103-2899

http://www.thoracic.theclinics.com

THORACIC SURGERY CLINICS Volume 27, Number 2
May 2017 ISSN 1547-4127, ISBN-13: 978-0-323-52862-7

Editor: John Vassallo (j.vassallo@elsevier.com)
Developmental Editor: Susan Showalter

Thoracic Surgery Clinics (ISSN 1547-4127) is published quarterly by Elsevier Inc., 360 Park Avenue South, New York, NY 10010-1710. Months of publication are February, May, August, and November. Business and editorial offices: 1600 John F. Kennedy Boulevard, Suite 1800, Philadelphia, PA 19103-2899. Periodicals postage paid at New York, NY, and additional mailing offices. Subscription prices are $359.00 per year (US individuals), $521.00 per year (US institutions), $100.00 per year (US Students), $439.00 per year (Canadian individuals), $674.00 per year (Canadian institutions), $225.00 per year (Canadian and international students), $470.00 per year (international individuals), and $674.00 per year (international institutions). Foreign air speed delivery is included in all Clinics' subscription prices. All prices are subject to change without notice. **POSTMASTER:** Send address changes to Thoracic Surgery Clinics, Elsevier Health Sciences Division, Subscription Customer Service, 3251 Riverport Lane, Maryland Heights, MO 63043. **Customer Service (orders, claims, online, change of address): Telephone: 1-800-654-2452 (U.S. and Canada); 314-447-8871 (outside U.S. and Canada). Fax: 314-447-8029. E-mail: journalscustomerservice-usa@elsevier.com (for print support); journalsonlinesupport-usa@elsevier.com (for online support).**

Reprints. For copies of 100 or more, of articles in this publication, please contact Commercial Rights Department, Elsevier Inc., 360 Park Avenue South, New York, NY 10010-1710. Tel: 212-633-3874; Fax: 212-633-3820; E-mail: reprints@elsevier.com.

Thoracic Surgery Clinics is covered in *MEDLINE/PubMed (Index Medicus), EMBASE/Excerpta Medica, Science Citation Index Expanded (SciSearch®), Journal Citation Reports/Science Edition,* and *Current Contents®/Clinical Medicine.*

Contributors

CONSULTING EDITOR

M. BLAIR MARSHALL, MD, FACS
Chief, Division of Thoracic Surgery, Associate
Professor, Department of Surgery,
Georgetown University Medical Center,
Georgetown University School of Medicine,
Washington, DC

EDITOR

HENNING A. GAISSERT, MD
Associate Professor of Surgery, Harvard
Medical School, Visiting Surgeon,
Massachusetts General Hospital, Boston,
Massachusetts

AUTHORS

EDWARD J. BERGERON, MD
Division of Cardiothoracic Surgery,
Department of Surgery, University of
Colorado, Anschutz Medical Campus, Aurora,
Colorado

WILLIAM BURFEIND Jr, MD
Chief, Department of Surgery, St. Luke's
University Health Network, Bethlehem,
Pennsylvania; Clinical Associate Professor of
Surgery, Temple University Medical School,
Philadelphia, Pennsylvania

ANTHONY CIPRIANO, MD
Resident, Department of Surgery, St. Luke's
University Health Network, Bethlehem,
Pennsylvania

SHARON L. CLANCY, MD
Division of Plastic Surgery, City of Hope,
Duarte, California

LORETTA J. ERHUNMWUNSEE, MD
Division of Thoracic Surgery, City of Hope,
Duarte, California

IRINA FELKER, PhD
Novosibirsk Tuberculosis Research Institute,
Federal State Budgetary Institution, Russian
Ministry of Health, Novosibirsk, Russian
Federation

FELIX G. FERNANDEZ, MD, MSc
Associate Professor, Section of General
Thoracic Surgery, Emory University School
of Medicine, Atlanta, Georgia

DAVID M. JABLONS, MD
Department of Thoracic Surgery, University
of California, San Francisco, San Francisco,
California

ONKAR V. KHULLAR, MD
Assistant Professor, Section of General
Thoracic Surgery, Emory University School
of Medicine, Atlanta, Georgia

DENIS KRASNOV, MD, PhD
Head, Department of Surgical, Novosibirsk
Tuberculosis Research Institute, Federal State
Budgetary Institution, Russian Ministry of
Health, Novosibirsk, Russian Federation

VLADIMIR KRASNOV, MD, PhD
Professor, Director, Novosibirsk Tuberculosis
Research Institute, Federal State Budgetary
Institution, Russian Ministry of Health,
Novosibirsk, Russian Federation

JOHANNES R. KRATZ, MD
Department of Thoracic Surgery, University of
California, San Francisco, San Francisco,
California

MICHAEL LANUTI, MD
Director of Thoracic Oncology, Division of
Thoracic Surgery, Massachusetts General
Hospital, Associate Professor of Surgery,
Harvard Medical School, Boston,
Massachusetts

PETER BJØRN LICHT, MD, PhD
Professor of Surgery, Department of
Cardiothoracic Surgery, Odense University
Hospital, Odense, Denmark

SARAH MAJERCIK, MD, MBA, FACS
Division of Trauma and Surgical Critical Care,
Intermountain Medical Center, Murray, Utah

ROBERT A. MEGUID, MD, MPH
Assistant Professor, Division of Cardiothoracic
Surgery, Department of Surgery, University of
Colorado, Anschutz Medical Campus, Aurora,
Colorado

ROBERT E. MERRITT, MD
Associate Professor, Director, Division of
Thoracic Surgery, The Ohio State University
Wexner Medical Center, Columbus, Ohio

JOHN D. MITCHELL, MD
Courtenay C. and Lucy Patten Davis Endowed
Chair in Thoracic Surgery, Professor and Chief,
Section of General Thoracic Surgery, Division
of Cardiothoracic Surgery, Department of
Surgery, University of Colorado School of
Medicine, Aurora, Colorado

FREDRIC M. PIERACCI, MD, MPH, FACS
Trauma Medical Director, Denver Health
Medical Center, Associate Professor of
Surgery, University of Colorado School of
Medicine, Denver, Colorado

HANS PILEGAARD, MD
Associate Professor of Surgery, Department of
Clinical Medicine, Aarhus University,

Department of Cardiothoracic and Vascular
Surgery, Aarhus University Hospital Skejby,
Aarhus N, Denmark

DAN J. RAZ, MD
Division of Thoracic Surgery, City of Hope,
Duarte, California

PAUL SCHIPPER, MD, FACS, FACCP
Professor of Surgery and Program Director,
Cardiothoracic Residency, Section of General
Thoracic Surgery, Division of Cardiothoracic
Surgery, Department of Surgery, Oregon
Health and Sciences University, Portland,
Oregon

BORIS SEPESI, MD, FACS
Assistant Professor, Department of Thoracic
and Cardiovascular Surgery, The University of
Texas MD Anderson Cancer Center, Houston,
Texas

K ROBERT SHEN, MD
Associate Professor of Surgery, Consultant,
Division of General Thoracic Surgery, Mayo
Clinic, Rochester, Minnesota

DMITRY SKVORTSOV, PhD
Thoracic Surgeon, Novosibirsk Tuberculosis
Research Institute, Federal State Budgetary
Institution, Russian Ministry of Health,
Novosibirsk, Russian Federation

MATHEW THOMAS, MD
Assistant Professor of Surgery, Consultant,
Division of Cardiothoracic Surgery, Mayo
Clinic, Jacksonville, Florida

BRANDON H. TIEU, MD, FACS
Assistant Professor of Surgery, Section of
General Thoracic Surgery, Division of
Cardiothoracic Surgery, Department of
Surgery, Oregon Health and Sciences
University, Portland, Oregon

GAVITT WOODARD, MD
Department of Surgery, University of California,
San Francisco, San Francisco, California

CAMERON D. WRIGHT, MD
Division of Thoracic Surgery, Massachusetts
General Hospital, Mathisen Family Professor of
Surgery, Harvard Medical School, Boston,
Massachusetts

Contents

have substantial benefit (decreased ventilator and intensive care unit days, improved pulmonary function, and improved long-term functional outcome) when they undergo surgery compared with nonoperative management.

Minimal Invasive Repair of Pectus Excavatum and Carinatum

Hans Pilegaard and Peter Bjørn Licht

Minimal invasive surgery has become the gold standard for surgical repair of pectus excavatum. The procedure can be performed as fast-track surgery and cosmetic results are excellent. In addition, cardiac performance improves after correction. With increased awareness on the Internet, the number of patients who seek help continues to rise, primarily for cosmetic reasons. Pectus carinatum is much less frequent than pectus excavatum. Over the past decade surgery has largely been replaced by compression techniques that use a brace, and cosmetic results are good. Rare combinations of pectus excavatum and carinatum may be treated by newer surgical methods.

Straight Back Syndrome

Cameron D. Wright

Straight back syndrome is a rare condition usually associated with mitral valve prolapse and "pseudo-heart disease" caused by a very narrow anterior-posterior chest due to the loss of the normal dorsal curvature of the thoracic spine. More rarely, the narrowed upper chest may compress the trachea causing extrinsic tracheal obstruction. If severe enough, this requires operative repair by effectively opening up the upper chest by a variety of techniques to allow the trachea enough room to avoid compression.

Management of Primary Soft Tissue Tumors of the Chest Wall

Anthony Cipriano and William Burfeind Jr

Primary chest wall tumors are rare and represent a challenging clinical entity. Preoperative work-up includes a thorough history, radiographic imaging, and a biopsy approach that does not make a future definitive resection more difficult. Treatment decisions are based on tumor histology, stage, local aggressiveness, and responsiveness to chemotherapy and radiation. Wide excision is the foundation of treatment of most malignant primary chest wall tumors. The role of radiation therapy in the neoadjuvant or adjuvant setting is to reduce local recurrence. The use of adjuvant chemotherapy is more controversial. For most primary chest wall malignancies, margin-negative resection remains the best chance of cure.

Management of Lung Cancer Invading the Superior Sulcus

Johannes R. Kratz, Gavitt Woodard, and David M. Jablons

Superior sulcus tumors have posed a formidable therapeutic challenge since their original description by Pancoast and Tobias in the early twentieth century. Initial therapeutic efforts with radiotherapy were associated with high rates of relapse and mortality. Bimodality therapy with complete surgical resection in the 1960s paved the way for trimodality therapy as the current standard of care in the treatment of superior sulcus tumors. The evolution of treatment approaches over time has provided outcomes that come increasingly closer to rivaling those of similarly staged nonapical lung cancer.

resection of lung cancer invading the chest wall, excluding the superior sulcus of the chest, is poorly defined. Survival of patients with lung cancer invading the chest wall is dependent on lymph node involvement and completeness of en-bloc resection. In some patients harboring T3N0 disease, 5-year survival in excess of 50% can be achieved. Offering en-bloc resection of lung cancer invading chest wall to patients with T3N1 or T3N2 disease is controversial.

Large chest wall resections can result in skeletal instability, altered respiratory mechanics, and significant cosmetic defects. Here the authors review a variety of prostheses that can be used to reconstruct these defects, the indications for their use, the technique for implantation, and the available data regarding their clinical outcomes.

THORACIC SURGERY CLINICS

THE CLINICS ARE AVAILABLE ONLINE!
Access your subscription at:
www.theclinics.com

Preface

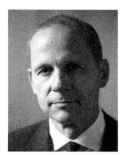

Henning A. Gaissert, MD
Editor

To be a specialist of rare disorders is a recurring challenge for the general thoracic surgeon. This age encourages the infinite expectation of perfection in those who seek our advice and, not least, in us. Chest wall disorders demand our attention because early diagnosis, complete resection, and durable, pain-free reconstruction are just as important to our patients as in the common diseases we treat, yet must be accomplished on a very narrow base of knowledge, experience, and evidence. For uncommon clinical problems of the chest wall, we more often find ourselves in need of silent study and our colleagues' collective wisdom. We are then fortunate to discover in this present collection reviews by experts to guide us in difficult clinical decisions. I owe a debt of gratitude to each contributor for including the pearls and pitfalls of clinical practice that enhance a review to the level of essential information. And when we emerge from silence in need of further communication, we know we find in each author a willing advisor; luck has it that even calls to Denmark and Russia remain affordable.

Henning A. Gaissert, MD
Massachusetts General Hospital
Harvard Medical School
Founders 7
55 Fruit Street
Boston, MA 02114, USA

E-mail address:
hgaissert@partners.org

Thorac Surg Clin 27 (2017) xi
http://dx.doi.org/10.1016/j.thorsurg.2017.02.001
1547-4127/17/© 2017 Published by Elsevier Inc.

Acute Chest Wall Infections
Surgical Site Infections, Necrotizing Soft Tissue Infections, and Sternoclavicular Joint Infection

Paul Schipper, MD*, Brandon H. Tieu, MD

KEYWORDS

- Surgical site infections • SSI • Wound infection • Necrotizing soft tissue infection
- Necrotizing fasciitis • Sternoclavicular joint infection • Sternoclavicular pyoarthrosis

KEY POINTS

- Posterolateral thoracotomy surgical site infections are uncommon and in most cases can be treated with a vacuum dressing.
- Sternoclavicular joint (SCJ) infections are uncommon and best treated with joint resection.
- There are several options for wound management and soft tissue coverage of a SCJ after resection.
- Necrotizing soft tissue infections of the chest occur most often after chest tube placement for an infectious etiology; favorable outcomes require a high index of suspicion and emergent surgical debridement.
- The signs and symptoms of a necrotizing soft tissue can be mimicked by more common postoperative sequelae, including postthoracotomy pain, subcutaneous emphysema, and soft tissue hematoma.

Acute infections of the chest wall are uncommon and those requiring surgical intervention are prone to misdiagnosis, overdiagnosis, and delayed diagnosis. This review discusses 3 distinct but related acute chest wall infections, and their pathology, diagnosis, and treatment: (1) surgical site infection (SSI) or wound infection of an anterior, lateral, or posterior thoracotomy, (2) necrotizing soft tissue infections of the thorax including necrotizing fasciitis, and (3) sternoclavicular joint (SCJ) infections or sternoclavicular pyoarthrosis. Infection and treatment of a median sternotomy wound is covered extensively in the literature and is not discussed in this review.

POSTOPERATIVE SURGICAL SITE INFECTION OF ANTERIOR, LATERAL, OR POSTERIOR THORACOTOMY

Whereas the treatment of thoracic SSIs, with a few exceptions discussed below, has not changed considerably in many years, the definition, tracking, risk stratification, and efforts at prevention of SSIs have become far more sophisticated. The General Thoracic Society of Thoracic Surgeons (STS) Database version 2.3 currently defines a SSI according to the Centers for Disease Control and Prevention definition, outlined in **Box 1**. Using these definitions, thoracic surgeons

Section of General Thoracic Surgery, Division of Cardiothoracic Surgery, Department of Surgery, Oregon Health and Sciences University, 3181 SW Sam Jackson Park Road L353, Portland, OR 97239, USA
* Corresponding author.
E-mail address: schippep@ohsu.edu

Thorac Surg Clin 27 (2017) 73–86
http://dx.doi.org/10.1016/j.thorsurg.2017.01.001
1547-4127/17/© 2017 Elsevier Inc. All rights reserved.

Box 1
Definitions of surgical site infections according to Centers for Disease Control and Prevention and the National Healthcare Safety Network and used by Society of Thoracic Surgeons General Thoracic Database

Superficial incisional SSI

Infection occurs within 30 days after the operative procedure *and* involves only skin and subcutaneous tissue of the incision *and* patient has at least 1 of the following:

1. Purulent drainage from the superficial incision;
2. Organisms isolated from an aseptically obtained culture of fluid or tissue from the superficial incision;
3. At least 1 of the following signs or symptoms of infection: pain or tenderness, localized swelling, redness, or heat, and superficial incision is deliberately opened by surgeon and is culture positive or not cultured (a culture-negative finding does not meet this criterion); and/or
4. Diagnosis of superficial incisional SSI by the surgeon or attending physician.

Deep incisional SSI

Infection occurs within 30 days after the operative procedure if no implant is left in place or within 1 year if implant is in place and infection seems to be related to the operative procedure *and* involves deep soft tissues (eg, fascial and muscle layers) of the incision *and* patient has at least 1 of the following:

1. Purulent drainage from the deep incision but not from the organ/space component of the surgical site;
2. A deep incision spontaneously dehisces or is deliberately opened by a surgeon and is culture positive or not cultured when the patient has at least 1 of the following signs or symptoms: fever (>38°C), or localized pain or tenderness (a culture-negative finding does not meet this criterion);
3. An abscess or other evidence of infection involving the deep incision is found on direct examination, during reoperation, or by histopathologic or radiologic examination; and/or
4. Diagnosis of a deep incisional SSI by a surgeon or attending physician.

Organ/space SSI

An organ/space SSI involves any part of the body, excluding the skin incision, fascia, or muscle layers, that is opened or manipulated during the operative procedure. An organ/space SSI must meet the following criterion:

Infection occurs within 30 days after the operative procedure if no implant is left in place or within 1 year if implant is in place and the infection seems to be related to the operative procedure *and* infection involves any part of the body, excluding the skin incision, fascia, or muscle layers, that is opened or manipulated during the operative procedure *and* patient has at least 1 of the following:

1. Purulent drainage from a drain that is placed through a stab wound into the organ/space;
2. Organisms isolated from an aseptically obtained culture of fluid or tissue in the organ/space;
3. An abscess or other evidence of infection involving the organ/space that is found on direct examination, during reoperation, or by histopathologic or radiologic examination; and/or
4. Diagnosis of an organ/space SSI by a surgeon or attending physician.

Abbreviation: SSI, surgical site infection.
Adapted from Horan TC, Andrus M, Dudeck MA. CDC/NHSN surveillance definition of health care-associated infection and criteria for specific types of infections in the acute care setting. Am J Infect Control 2008;36:313–4; with permission.

reporting to the STS database between January 2013 and December 2015 report a relatively low rate of SSI related to common thoracic procedures (**Table 1**).

Risk factors for a SSI include extremes of age, poor nutritional status, diabetes, smoking, obesity, coexistent infections at remote body site, colonization of skin or gastrointestinal tract with microorganisms, altered immune response, duration of hospital preoperative stay, duration of surgical scrub, quality of skin antisepsis for surgical team, preoperative shaving, preoperative skin preparation, duration of operation, appropriate antimicrobial prophylaxis, operating room ventilation, instrument

Table 1
Surgical site infections by depth of common thoracic procedures reported to Society of Thoracic Surgeons General Thoracic Database, January 2013 to December 2015

	N	Superficial (%)	Deep (%)	Organ/Space (%)
Segmentectomy	3400	0.2	0.1	0
Lobectomy	30,422	0.6	0.1	0.2
Pneumonectomy	1484	1.2	0.3	0.7
Decortication	13,117	0.6	0.1	0.2

sterilization, foreign material in the surgical site, surgical drains, and surgical technique. It is clear from this list that many risk factors are modifiable, some are not, and some are unavoidable within the time constraints of urgent or emergent surgery.[1,2]

Current and comprehensive recommendations for SSI prevention can be found in reviews by Young and Khadaroo[2] from 2014, Alexander and colleagues[3] from 2011 and from the Centers for Disease Control and Prevention at www.cdc.gov/ncidod/dhqp/nhsn.html.

SMOKING CESSATION AND SURGICAL SITE INFECTIONS

Smoking increases the risk of complications after thoracic surgery. Smoking increases wound infection rates through several mechanisms, including vasoconstriction and decreased tissue P_{O_2}.[4] This increased risk of SSI can be mitigated 4 weeks after smoking cessation. Unfortunately, the other risks associated with undergoing surgery as a current or recent smoker take longer to subside after cessation. In the STS General Thoracic database, current smokers compared with never smokers undergoing resection for lung cancer between 1999 and 2007 had a higher risk-adjusted odds ratio of death of 3.5 ($P = .03$). Quitting reduced the risk of death, but this occurred slowly over time and remained statistically similar when groups who had quit less than 2 weeks, 2 to 4 weeks, and 4 weeks to 1 year were compared. A similar slow mitigation of risk after smoking cessation was also found for pulmonary morbidity.[5] Two additional STS General Thoracic database reports from 2002 to 2009 and 2012 to 2014 showed that cigarette smoking increased major morbidity (including tracheostomy, reintubation, initial ventilator support longer than 48 hours, adult respiratory distress syndrome, bronchopleural fistula, pulmonary embolus, pneumonia, unexpected return to the operating room, bleeding requiring reoperation, and myocardial infarction) by 60% over never smokers after lung resection. However, neither study showed a difference in mortality between smokers and never smokers.[6,7] Finally, the STS data confirmed the findings by Barrera and colleagues[8] that, contrary to previous reports, there is no increased risk of morbidity for lung resection immediately after smoking cessation (0–4 weeks).[9]

The risk reduction of SSI with smoking cessation before surgery seems to occur immediately and represents a true modifiable risk factor. A randomized, controlled trial in 2003 placed small incisions on the buttocks of healthy volunteers (smokers and nonsmokers) and randomized the smokers to 1 of 3 groups: (1) continue smoking 1 pack per day, (2) quitting, or (3) quitting with nicotine replacement. The wounds were made after the first week of smoking with subsequent wounds made at 4, 8, and 12 weeks after randomization. The wound infection rate was 12% in smokers compared with 2% in never smokers ($P<.05$). The wound infection rate in previous smokers randomized to either abstinence group (nicotine replacement or not) was 1% after 4 weeks and remained low at 8 and 12 weeks.[10] The conclusion of this randomized study is that smoking increases the risk of wound infection; however, this risk is negated with quitting for 4 weeks either with or without nicotine replacement. Three previous studies have shown a similar reduction in wound infection rates with 4 weeks of smoking cessation, but none of these studies included chest incisions.[11–13]

A preoperative visit, especially to discuss lung cancer surgery, represents an opportunity to teach behavior modification strategies that encourages smoking cessation. Although the immediate benefits for a planned surgical procedure may be limited to a reduction in wound infection risk, the long-term benefit for the patient's health is much greater.

TREATMENT OF SUPERFICIAL SURGICAL SITE INFECTION

Ironically, the treatment of a thoracic superficial SSI is part of its definition: drainage. A cellulitis can be treated with antibiotics alone. Any purulence requires source control by opening the skin and underlying fat wide enough to allow adequate drainage. The wound, in particular the muscle layers, should be inspected for evidence of infection originating from deeper tissue layers. If a deep tissue infection is present, that requires debridement and drainage as well. The wound can then be treated with wet to dry dressings or negative pressure wound therapy until closed by secondary intention.

TREATMENT OF DEEP SURGICAL SITE INFECTIONS OF THE THORAX

By definition, a deep SSI of the thorax has penetrated or involves 1 or more of the muscle layers—latissimus dorsi muscle, serratus anterior muscle, or less likely the rhomboids, trapezius, or pectoralis major or minor. These muscles are generally well-perfused and resistant to infection. They are often sacrificed as functional muscles and transferred to other parts of the body as muscle flaps to impart their tremendous ability to resist infection and heal wounds. In addition, adequate drainage of the superficial component of a deep thoracic SSI may be enough to allow systemic antibiotics and the surrounding muscle to clear the infection. Several anatomic factors of the deep tissue spaces of the chest wall are challenging for the treating surgeon.

1. The scapula–thoracic articulation—the upper extremity articulates with the thorax in large part through the scapula–thoracic articulation. This is described in the section on SCJ infections. In brief, there is a relatively open space under the scapula, allowing the scapula to slide on the chest wall. The scapula is both moved and held in place by several large muscle groups, including the serratus anterior, latissimus dorsi, and rhomboids. All of these muscles have a relatively open space, with at most loose connective tissue deep between them and the underlying rib/intercostal muscle to accommodate the movement of the scapula. By comparison, the pectoralis major muscle is inserted broadly on the ribs and sternum across the anterior chest wall that eliminates this space. A deep tissue infection may potentially spread easily through the scapula–thoracic articulation, without necessarily involving the structures surrounding the space. Alternatively, a surgeon opening a wound may find a large space that is not infected, but now must decide whether or not to pack yards of gauze into the scapula–thoracic articulation.
2. Anterior and posterior muscle-sparing thoracotomies do not divide the muscle body, insertion, or origin of the large muscles of the chest wall (serratus anterior, latissimus dorsi, rhomboids),

but mobilizes them to gain access to an interspace. This can leave large, open, connected planes in the chest wall that create similar issues to the scapula–thoracic articulation.
3. Many methods of closing both thoracoscopy and thoracotomy incisions do not close the intercostal space, or do not close it to an "air-tight" seal. Rather, this closure relies on the overlying soft tissue of the deep space to seal the pleural space. Once the deep layers of the chest wall are opened, the wound is essentially opened into the organ space and may represent a "sucking chest wound." In addition, once a thoracic deep SSI has developed, there may be no anatomic barrier separating the organ space from the infected deep tissue layer.

These 3 issues mean that once the deeper layers are opened, even in a minimal fashion, the wound can rapidly involve a considerable amount of the chest wall and/or the organ space.

The first principle is to drain all areas of infection, while minimizing the spread by extending the dissection into uninfected tissue planes. After the infection has been adequately drained and debrided, dressing changes should occur between 1 and 4 times per day using gauze that has been soaked in saline or another solution (eg, Dakin's solution). Because of the complexity of thoracoscopy and thoracotomy wounds, their depth, and multiple tissue layers, the principle of using 1 piece of gauze to pack the wound is important. This practice prevents orphaned and forgotten wound dressings from being incorporated into the wound only to cause lingering infections. To accommodate a large space or multiple areas that require packing, several rolled gauze dressings can be tied together to ensure complete removal with each dressing change. Although tempting, it is usually unnecessary to pack large volumes of dressing into the scapula–thoracic articulation. Once the initial opening and drainage is found to be sufficient on reinspection, a vacuum dressing can be used to manage the complexities of an open thoracotomy or thoracoscopy incision.

TREATMENT OF ORGAN/SPACE SURGICAL SITE INFECTIONS

In the thorax, treatment of an organ space infection means treatment of empyema, mediastinitis, osteomyelitis of rib or vertebral body, postpneumonectomy empyema, and postlobectomy empyema with or without bronchopleural fistula. Some infections originate in the organ/space such as pneumonia to parapneumonic empyema, perforated viscus, anastomotic leak, and infected reconstruction of a chest wall resection (mesh). Source control would involve identifying and addressing these sources. Other infections spread from a more superficial SSI to involve the organ space. In this case, it is almost always some version of an empyema. Once a more dangerous source is ruled out (bronchopleural fistula, esophageal perforation, anastomotic leak, or pneumonia), source control can be obtained with chest tube drainage, escalating to thoracoscopy and deloculation, thoracotomy and deloculation, or window thoracostomy as needed. Broad-spectrum antibiotic coverage is initiated based on the suspected source—skin flora, oral flora, or gastrointestinal tract—and narrowed as culture data become available.

NEGATIVE PRESSURE WOUND THERAPY AND VACUUM-ASSISTED CLOSURE

Many of the complexities of a SSI of a chest incision can be managed with a vacuum dressing. Vacuum-assisted closure (VAC) was first described in 1993 as a method to improve healing and wound debridement of open fractures.[14] Vacuum dressings have been used effectively for many years with superficial wounds (skin and subcutaneous fat), including infected wounds.[15] A commercially available vacuum pump was introduced in 1995. In 2005, VAC was used in conjunction with standard organ space therapies to treat deep soft tissue infections of the chest wall: empyema necessitans, postresection empyema with deep SSI, and trauma with superficial, deep, and organ space infections.[16] The treatment of deep organ space infection (empyema) with VAC and open window thoracostomy (OWT) was first reported in 2006.[17] In the decade since, multiple short case series have reported using VAC to treat increasingly complex variations of organ space infection (parapneumonic empyema, postresection empyema, and empyema with and without bronchopleural fistula). No randomized, controlled trials have been done comparing vacuum therapy with the more traditional wet to dry dressing therapies for thoracic wounds. The proposed benefits of the VAC include portability to allow patient mobilization and activity, reduced costs compared with conventional wound treatment,[18] ease of application, VAC changes that can be done at the bedside or as an outpatient, and facilitation of early discharge.

Negative pressure wound therapy seems to work through multiple mechanisms. In animal studies, with a negative pressure of 125 mm Hg, the blood flow to treated areas is increased 4-fold from baseline. Granulation tissue formation was significantly higher with both continuous and intermittent negative pressure, and tissue bacterial counts were reduced.[19] These animal study findings were confirmed in human use with enhanced granulation tissue formation, removal of exudates, edema reduction, increased tissue perfusion, and wound volume reduction.[20]

Because there are many variations on thoracic SSIs, especially when the infection originates from, may spread into, or already has spread into the organ space, the treatment of a SSI with a VAC is informed by the following questions:

1. Can a vacuum dressing be used to manage a deep SSI of a thoracotomy incision?
2. How are chest drains managed in conjunction with a vacuum dressing?
3. Can a vacuum dressing be used in a window thoracostomy?
4. Can a vacuum dressing be placed on the lung?
5. Can a vacuum dressing be placed on the mediastinum/bronchial stump?

Can a Vacuum Dressing Be Used to Manage a Deep Surgical Site Infection of a Thoracotomy Incision?

Successful management of deep thoracotomy SSIs has been reported in case reports and case series. Welvaart and colleagues[21] described the use of a VAC after dehiscence of a right posterolateral thoracotomy for resection of a superior sulcus tumor. The patient had received neoadjuvant chemoradiotherapy with cisplatin/etoposide and 46 Gy of radiation. Six weeks later, the patient underwent a successful resection and was discharged home on postoperative day 7. The patient returned on postoperative day 27 with a wound dehiscence and a hydropneumothorax. After initial treatment of the hydropneumothorax with a chest tube and wound coverage with an occlusive dressing, a vacuum dressing was placed on the deep wound with suction applied at 50 mm Hg on postoperative day 29. The vacuum dressing was changed every 72 hours by a home care nurse and after 8 weeks the wound was completely healed.

O'Connor and colleagues[16] showed that complex chest wounds, including thoracotomy incisions, could be managed successfully with a VAC. Their case series of 17 patients from 2000 to 2003 were broken into 2 groups. Group 1 had primary chest wall processes: 4 with necrotizing soft tissue infections and 3 with penetrating chest traumas and tissue loss. Group 2 consisted of 10 patients with empyema. Six had parapneumonic infections that included 3 with empyema necessitans and 4 with postoperative empyemas. After extensive debridement of the infected and necrotic soft tissue and decortication for the empyemas, vacuum dressings were applied to all the wounds. The average wound size was 16 × 7 cm. The wound vacuum systems were changed every 2 days and the average duration of vacuum dressing usage was 9 days (range, 3–21). In group 1, final wound closure was established with delayed primary closure in 4 patients, split thickness skin graft in 2, and 1 patient healed by secondary intention. In group 2, 4 patients had advancement muscle flaps with delayed primary closures of their wounds. Two had split thickness skin grafts and 2 healed by delayed primary closures. The remaining 2 healed by secondary intention.

How Are Chest Drains Managed in Conjunction with a Vacuum Dressing?

There are few data to guide the management of chest drains in conjunction with negative pressure vacuum dressings. All the chest tubes in the series from O'Connor and associates were managed with a standard protocol for thoracotomy patients; however, the protocol was not described in the article. The investigators reported that the drain management was not influenced by the vacuum dressing. It must be noted that all their patients had closed chest walls where the drains and vacuum dressings were not functioning in the same closed space. The physiology of competitive suction resulting in a net neutral suction (eg, chest tube pulling fluid in 1 direction while vacuum dressing pulling it in a different direction) has been reported in median sternotomy wounds with resulting undrained fluid collections.[22] This occurrence has not been reported in posterior lateral thoracotomy wounds, but the vacuum dressing has been used to treat subcutaneous emphysema.

Can a Vacuum Dressing Be Used in a Window Thoracostomy?

In 2006, Varker and Ng[17] reported the first use of the VAC to treat an open empyema cavity. The patient developed an empyema without a bronchopleural fistula 3 months after a right lower lobectomy with chest wall resection and reconstruction with a 2-mm expanded polytetrafluoroethylene mesh. After debriding the wound and packing the open pleural space for a few days, a vacuum dressing was applied. The patient was discharged home 2 weeks later and after 4 months the wound was completely healed. Since that first report, other case series have reported the use of the vacuum dressing with OWT.[17,23,24] Palmen and colleagues[24] treated 11 patients with OWT successfully using VAC. The foam was packed directly onto the lung, even in the setting of

alveolopleural fistulae from decortication, and filled the pleural space. All the VAC patients had the OWT closed within 1 month of starting the vacuum therapy either with the aid of muscular transposition flaps (n = 9) or by secondary intention (n = 2). The investigators proposed an additional advantage that the negative pressure dressing improves expansion of the consolidated lung parenchyma. Begum and Papagiannopoulos[23] reported similar outcomes in 10 patients with empyema and OTW. The VAC was placed at the time of open drainage and debridement or on postoperative day 1. The VAC therapy allowed early rehabilitation and return to activities of daily living. None of the wounds required surgical closure. A recent review evaluating the use of VAC for pleural space infections concluded that the VAC, as an adjunct to standard therapy, could potentially reduce inpatient length of treatment and morbidity.[25] Recently a min-VAC therapy system has been introduced.[26] In patients with poor performance status (Karnofsky index of ≤50%) who cannot tolerate a standard thoracotomy and decortication, a small, 5- to 6-cm thoracotomy incision is created and a Alexis (Applied Medical, Rancho Santa Margarita, CA) wound protector retractor is inserted. After local debridement and drainage of the pleural space, the standard foam dressing is inserted with the initial suction set to −75 mm Hg. Other researchers have advanced this technique by adding the VAC instill pad over the dressing. The vacuum device has an automated delivery system that can regulate a predetermined volume of 0.02% polyhexanide solution. This process allows for pleural decontamination with irrigation and removal of infectious materials.[27]

Can a Vacuum Dressing Be Placed on the Lung?

There is a paucity of reports that have addressed this aspect of VAC therapy. Varker and Ng[17] placed the VAC dressing only after several days of saline dressing changes and the development of granulation tissue. All of the patients in the series from O'Connor and coworkers had closed chest walls and, therefore, none of the vacuum sponges were in direct contact with the pleural space or lung. Palmen and colleagues[24] placed the polyurethane foam directly onto the lung and reported no issues with bleeding or parenchymal damage with application of the −125 mm Hg. Even patients that had alveolopleural fistulas had the polyurethane foam directly placed on the parenchyma without adverse effects and demonstrated resolution of the air leaks with the VAC dressing. Begum and Papagiannopoulos[23] covered the lung with a nonadherent silicone membrane before placement of the foam sponge with a negative pressure of −100 mm Hg. Once again, no VAC-related complications were noted.[16,17,23,24]

Can a Vacuum Dressing Be Placed on the Mediastinum/Bronchial Stump?

The VAC dressing has been used to manage post-lobectomy and postpneumonectomy spaces next to the mediastinum and bronchial stumps. Saadi and colleagues[28] treated 27 patients with complex intrathoracic infections with VAC dressings and closed chest walls rather than OWT. They placed sterile gauze pads on the mediastinum before the foam placement. Patients with bronchopleural fistula and empyemas after gastrointestinal perforation or anastomotic leaks had the VAC placed over the gauze-covered mediastinal structures after source control with primary repair, with or without flap coverage, or esophageal exclusion. VAC pressures ranging from −50 to −75 mm Hg were used in this study. The investigators reported only 1 VAC-related complication of bleeding from the mammary vein requiring surgical intervention. A series of patients reported by Groetzner and colleagues[29] that included empyemas, postlobectomy empyemas, and postpneumonectomy empyemas, placed the polyvinyl-alcohol foam (White Foam) next to the mediastinal structures and filled the remaining pleural space with the standard polyurethane foam. They included patients with bronchopleural fistulas after bronchial stump closure and buttressing with a muscle flap. The negative pressure setting were started at −75 mm Hg and increased to −125 mm Hg as healing progressed. They reported no VAC-related complication with this technique.

NECROTIZING SOFT TISSUE INFECTION

Necrotizing soft tissue infections that originate from or only involve the thorax are very uncommon. Before 2002, there were 15 published reports (1973–1998) with 47% showing a delay in diagnosis and a 67% mortality rate.[30] From 1999 to 2011, an additional 7 cases were reported. Necrotizing fasciitis that originates elsewhere (most often extremities) and spreads to the trunk is more common.[31] Successful treatment of a true necrotizing soft tissue infection mandates urgent surgical debridement. Approximately 90% of the reported necrotizing soft tissue infections of the thorax are found or evolve from the treatment of other thoracic pathologies, especially chest tube placement for empyema. Symptoms of necrotizing soft tissue infections are erythema, pain or tenderness beyond the margins of erythema, swelling, crepitance, and induration, with later findings including necrosis and skin bullae. Signs of systemic toxicity include hypotension, diaphoresis, fever, and anxiety. Historically, the diagnosis is delayed and many of the diagnostic signs and symptoms overlap with common findings after thoracic surgery, making a false-positive diagnosis a risk owing to the low pretest probability of disease.

Necrotizing soft tissue infections can be classified by the depth of necrosis or layer(s) involved: necrotizing adipositis (most common), necrotizing fasciitis, and necrotizing myositis. It is important to recognize that necrotizing fasciitis may be just 1 component of a multilayer necrotizing soft tissue infection. Necrotizing soft tissue infections can also be categorized by the causative organism (**Table 2**).

Although examples of the most common culprit organisms are given in **Table 2**, almost every known organism, either alone or in collaboration, has been implicated in causing a necrotizing soft tissue infection. A polymicrobial or synergistic necrotizing soft tissue infection is a slower process, may take days to develop, and usually follows gastrointestinal contamination of the subcutaneous planes with polymicrobial inoculation (perforated esophagus, gastric conduit, or esophagectomy anastomotic leak with chest tube drainage).

Table 2 Necrotizing soft tissue infections categorized by causative organism	
Polymicrobial or synergistic	Mixed anaerobes and aerobes, often bowel flora derived
Monomicrobial—1 very virulent organism	Usually beta hemolytic streptococcus
Water associated—seafood ingestion or injury contaminated by sea water	*Vibrio vulnificus* or *V damselae* Gram-negative marine related organisms
Fungal	Candida spp., Zygomycetes in an immunocompromised host

Adapted from Morgan M. Diagnosis and management of necrotising fasciitis: a multiparametric approach. J Hosp Infect 2010;75:250; with permission.

Monomicrobial necrotizing soft tissue infections involve an organism with a virulence factor that allows immune system evasion or quickens egress through tissue planes.[32] Water-associated necrotizing soft tissue infections result from an injury that is contaminated with warm sea water harboring *vibrio* species and is more common in the warm coastal areas of Asia.

In all necrotizing soft tissue infections, a cycle is established where the host immune system is overwhelmed in a localized area, the tissue becomes ischemic, the small vessels thrombose, and eventually the overlying tissue necrotizes. This thrombosis is caused by a localized hypercoagulable state, platelet–neutrophil plugging of vessels, and increased interstitial pressure from edema. A significant number of dermal capillaries must be compromised before skin necrosis occurs. The extent of infection and relative tissue ischemia often extends beyond any visible skin changes. If anaerobes are present, gases such as hydrogen, nitrogen, hydrogen sulfide, and methane are produced. These gases are not very soluble in water and produce crepitance. The relative ischemia inhibits polymorphonuclear cell oxidative destruction of bacteria and inhibits the penetration of blood born antibiotics into the infected tissue. Ischemia to nerves initially causes pain out of proportion to other findings and then, as the nerve dies, anesthesia. The dermis and epidermis are relatively resistant to tissue ischemia, and blistering followed by skin death are late findings.

DIAGNOSIS AND TREATMENT

Necrotizing soft tissue infections must be treated with surgical debridement if the patient is to survive. The reasons for this are implicit in the pathology. In a localized area, the immune system has been overwhelmed, medical therapy consisting of antibiotics cannot reach the offending organisms, and a domino effect occurs, where the infection progresses rapidly. The surgeon's role is vitally important and involves the following. First, determine that a necrotizing infection is present and not an alternative diagnosis of nonnecrotizing infection that may respond very well to antibiotics alone. Second, determine this early in the disease process so that morbidity and mortality are minimized or avoided. Finally, once the diagnosis is suspected, the extent of debridement requires resection of all necrotic tissue so that the host immune system and systemic antibiotics can salvage the situation.

Classically, necrotizing soft tissue infections are diagnosed clinically by pain, swelling, and erythema. A consistent feature is pain out of proportion to the swelling and with extension into areas that do not seem to be involved (painful early ischemia of nerves). Crepitance, skin blistering, and necrosis are late findings, so if they are present it strongly supports the diagnosis. However, if they are absent it should not exclude the diagnosis. Marks on the skin separately defining areas of erythema, edema, and tenderness can be closely observed (every 2–4 hours). Any progression or any doubt should result in a 1-cm^3 deep tissue biopsy with frozen section. The pathologist gains the most information with a biopsy from the interface between live and dead tissue. Pathology will be looking for superficial epidermal hyaline necrosis, dermal edema, polymorphonuclear infiltration into the dermis, inflammation and thrombosis of penetrating fascial vessels, and finally tissue necrosis.[33] In a necrotizing soft tissue infection, the surgeon will variably experience a foul smell (hydrogen sulfide from anaerobes) and see dishwater discharge (formed from necrosed polymorphonuclear cells and edema), a lack of bleeding (small vessel necrosis), a lack of muscle contraction (skeletal muscle ischemia and myonecrosis), and finally an "easy" separation of fascial planes. This final sign, "easy" separation of fascial planes, can be applied as a strong indicator of necrotizing fasciitis in the extremities and abdomen as the finger test. A 1- to 2-cm incision is made down to the fascia and blunt finger dissection is used to separate the planes. Easy passage of the finger is a positive test. This test is not as useful for necrotizing soft tissue infections of the chest wall. Thoracic surgeons are familiar with how easily a finger or hand can be passed under the scapula, latissimus muscle, serratus muscle, and some parts of the pectoralis muscle in a normal patient to separate the fascial planes. In addition, pleural fluid, blood, and subcutaneous emphysema can track along these planes without indicating the presence of a necrotizing soft tissue infection.

The most important determinant of mortality is timing and adequacy of initial debridement. Once a necrotizing soft tissue infection is confirmed, the boundaries of the debridement should be as wide as necessary to obtain healthy, bleeding tissue—skin, fat, and muscle. Debridement should continue every 12 to 36 hours until no further spread is seen. Tissue cultures from the affected areas (not swabs of blistering skin or bullae) should be obtained at each debridement and used to refine antibiotic therapy. Debridement can be massive; therefore, involving a plastic surgeon early in the process allows for planning for future soft tissue coverage.

Hyperbaric oxygen can be used as an adjunct to treatment of necrotizing soft tissue infections, especially in regard to wound healing. Unfortunately, it is not widely available, but has been and continues to be studied.[34,35] Hyperbaric oxygen as a therapy does not supersede early identification and surgical debridement in improving mortality and morbidity. Neutrophils use the partial pressure of oxygen in tissue to form oxygen free radicals to kill bacteria. By increasing the P_{O_2}, either nominally through increasing F_{IO_2} at atmospheric pressures or in a significant way with hyperbaric oxygen, the neutrophil bacterial kill rate can be increased.

STERNOCLAVICULAR JOINT INFECTION

Infection of the SCJ is uncommon, with fewer than 250 cases reported in the literature over the last 50 years. Because of the proximity of the SCJ to the great vessels and because treatment often involves debridement or resection in an inflamed and hostile arena, thoracic surgeons are called on to treat an unfamiliar disease process (septic arthritis) in a very familiar anatomy. Despite its rarity in the published literature, a thoracic surgery practice is likely to see a dozen or more cases over a career. The literature on the topic comes only from case series. No randomized trials have evaluated treatment decisions (surgical vs not, type of debridement) and because of the rarity of the infection, these trials are unlikely to occur. With this in mind, this review covers the diagnosis of this infection and attempts to answer the following questions.

1. Why is this joint predisposed to infections and what is the potential loss of function from removing the SCJ?
2. Does treatment of an infected joint require debridement or resection, or can antibiotic therapy alone or in combination with drainage suffice?
3. Once the joint is removed, what is the optimal method of closing the defect?

DIAGNOSIS

Most patients with an infected SCJ present with chest pain localized to the SCJ (78%) and can also complain of shoulder pain (25%) and rarely neck pain (2%). Rarely, is it just painless swelling (4%).[36] Tenderness of the joint (it hurts when you push on it) is present 90% of the time and may serve as the single most reliable diagnostic test. Unlike the typical presentation of septic arthritis that occurs shortly after onset of infection, the median duration of symptoms in a SCJ infection before presentation is 14 days. Fever and/or an increased white blood cell occur in one-half of patients.

Plain radiographs, computed tomography, or MRI are all used to evaluate the joint. Positive findings include widening of the joint space, joint destruction, and osteomyelitis of the clavicle, manubrium, or first rib. Because of its unique anatomy, the SCJ can seem to have irregular articular surfaces and a weathered appearance on computed tomography and MRI, compared with other joints. Older joints can become calcified and even sclerose. As a thoracic surgeon, you will look at many computed tomography scans with normal SCJs and you should familiarize yourself with the range of normal. If a unilateral infected joint is suspected clinically, the suspect joint can be compared radiographically to the contralateral joint. Evidence of a soft tissue infection around the joint swelling, streaking, phlegmon, or abscess can suggest joint involvement, but needs to be separated from a true joint infection. The soft tissue component often responds very well to antibiotic therapy alone, whereas a joint infection or abscess needs drainage and/or debridement. Imaging evidence of osteomyelitis in the clavicle, manubrium, or first rib is a strong indicator that joint resection or extensive debridement is required as opposed to incision and drainage or antibiotics alone.

Why Is This Joint Predisposed to Infections and What Is the Potential Loss of Function from Removing the Sternoclavicular Joint?

Although the SCJ is the only bony articulation between the upper extremity and the axial skeleton, there are many soft tissue structures, including the pectoralis major and minor muscles, latissimus dorsi muscle, rhomboid muscle, serratus anterior muscle, levator scapulae muscle, and trapezius muscle, that provide support and attachment, and allow for a profound mobility of the upper extremity on the axial skeleton. The true attachment of the scapula to the axial skeleton is the scapulothoracic articulation formed by all these muscles.

The SCJ is a diarthrodial (meaning freely movable) saddle joint with a synovial lining. It has a joint disc that is attached to the posterior capsule and this disc often has perforations. The blood supply comes from a vascular arcade off the internal mammary artery. In some cases, branches of the thyrocervical trunk perfuse the intraarticular disc. Unlike most diarthrodial joints, such as the knee, hip, or shoulder, the SCJ is lined by fibrocartilage, not hyaline cartilage. The presence of this bulky central disc may be the reason the SCJ seems to have the same susceptibility to infection as amphiarthrodial joints. These are joints with limited motion and without a synovial lining where bones are joined by fibrocartilage. Examples of these are the pubic symphysis, sacroiliac, and vertebral body joints. With aging, the amphiarthrodial joints tend to fuse, which may protect older patients from infection owing to sclerosis.

The SCJ involves the union of 3 bones that attach the first rib and manubrium to the head of the clavicle with an anterior and posterior joint capsule. The clavicle sweeps posterior from the SCJ to attach to the scapula at the acromioclavicular joint. The clavicle is fixed to the first rib by the costoclavicular ligament. The primary function of the clavicle can be thought of as a strut, keeping the scapula at a fixed distance from the axial skeleton. This allows muscles that attach to the axial skeleton and insert across the scapula into the humerus (such as the pectoralis major or latissimus dorsi) to obtain a lever arm and improves their function. If the joint is removed, the presence of the costoclavicular ligament, which attaches the clavicle to the first rib, can maintain this strut function.[37] Acus and colleagues[38] reported that a majority of patients in their series had little to no pain, weakness, or detriment to their range of motion after the excision of an average of 2.9 cm (and as much as 4 cm) of the medial clavicle; however, their series was not limited to SCJ resection for infection. Two surgical series involving 7 and 21 en bloc joint resections followed patients for a median of 2 years and asked them to rate their level of function by using a 3-point scale and reporting their range of motion, respectively. Results showed 100% of patients reported their function as "normal"[39] and "without limitations in range of motion."[40–42] In 2016, Kachala and colleagues[43] reported their 20-year experience with joint resection using a validated questionnaire of upper extremity function called QuickDASH. The scale extends from 0 to 100 with no impairment ranging 0 to 25 and mild impairment 25 to 50. Preresection scores were a mean of 10. Postresection scores were a mean of 19 ± 4 for muscle flap repair and 20 ± 8 for VAC. In summary, as long as the costoclavicular ligament is left intact, the SJC can be removed with no or very little change in upper extremity function.

In general, septic arthritis occurs in older patients (mean age of 65 years).[44] SCJ infections, however, occur in younger patients (mean age of 45 years) and when associated with intravenous (IV) drug use occurs even younger patients (mean age of 35 years). This resembles the amphiarthrodial or fibrous joint such as the sacroiliac joint (mean age of infected joint 22 years) and pubic symphysis (mean age of 48 years). Ross and Shamsuddin[44] postulate that the presence of the fibrous intraarticular disc, the 2 compartments it creates, and the more limited range of motion cause this joint to have the same susceptibility to bacterial infection as amphiarthrodial joints. With bacteremia, all joints are seeded with bacteria but the SCJ cannot clear the bacteria as efficiently.

In a metaanalysis, Ross and Shamsuddin[44] reviewed the published literature of SCJ infections from 1970 through 2003 and reported on 170 cases. Of these, 23% occurred with no predisposing condition, 21% with IV drug use, 24% with distant infection including central line, and 13% with diabetes. Less common were chronic renal failure, alcoholism, cirrhosis, and human immunodeficiency virus infection.[44] Since that time, clinicians have cited similar predisposing conditions with variability among the most common risk factors and related to the particular population the author served. Septic arthritis affects the SCJ in the general population 1% of the time, but this increases to 17% in IV drug users.[44] It is proposed that the increase is owing to the common use of the upper extremity for IV drug injection and with the development of subclavian vein thrombophlebitis, it can easily extend into the closely approximated joint. Another less likely explanation is the direct injection of the joint owing to a misdirected neck injection. Surgeons should be wary of needle fragments in an infected joint during debridement.

Clinically, this means that an SCJ infection should be suspected over other joints in a younger group of patients, and the other amphiarthrodial joints, such as the vertebral body, pubic symphysis, and sacroiliac joints should be considered when an SCJ infection is discovered.

Does Treatment of an Infected Joint Require Debridement or Resection, or Can Antibiotic Therapy Alone Suffice?

The treatment of any infected joint requires antibiotics and drainage. For reasons unknown and discussed, the SCJ seems to be unable to clear reliably even a minimal bacterial load despite IV antibiotics. Because of its rarity, no randomized trials exist comparing therapies with antibiotics alone or among the various methods of surgical therapy, including drainage alone, limited debridement, larger debridement, wide resection of the joint, and the methods of closure. Ross and Shamsuddin[44] summarized the reported therapies in their metaanalysis. Forty-two percent were only treated medically and 58% required surgery. Thirty-one percent underwent surgical debridement and 27% had an en bloc resection. Of the surgically treated patients, 10% (11 of 102) represented failure of medical therapy with escalation to surgical debridement and 24% (13 of 54) of the en bloc resections represented limited debridement failure escalated to en bloc resection.[45] Because complete removal of the joint has the greatest chance to resolve the infection and the unilateral loss of the SJC results in minimal to no loss of function, most authors have advocated for quick or immediate escalation of therapy to resection of the joint once infection is confirmed. **Figs. 1** and **2** illustrate en bloc resection of the SCJ.

The following statements should be considered when deciding the appropriate therapy for SCJ infections.

1. If the joint is not involved, it does not need to be drained or resected. Soft tissue infection such as a thrombophlebitis or chest wall cellulitis or myositis will respond well to appropriate medical therapy alone.
2. If there is a question as to joint involvement, aspiration can be attempted. A positive result would confirm a joint infection; however, owing to the small size of the joint space, aspiration is often nondiagnostic or is falsely negative.
3. If there is bone involvement—osteomyelitis, bone destruction—the joint will need to be removed either by extensive debridement or en bloc resection. Incision and drainage is inadequate.

Once the Joint Is Removed, What Is the Optimal Method of Closing the Defect?

This question has not been answered definitively. The options for closure are the same as with all surgical wounds and tissue defects created in

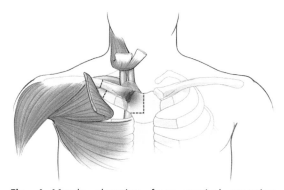

Fig. 1. Muscle elevation from surgical resection shows the sternal and clavicular heads of the sternocleidomastoid muscle being elevated off their insertion. The superomedial aspect of the pectoralis is also reflected. (*Reprinted from* Kachala S, D'Souza DM, Teixeira-Johnson L, et al. Surgical management of sternoclavicular joint infections. Ann Thorac Surg 2016;101:2155–60; with permission.)

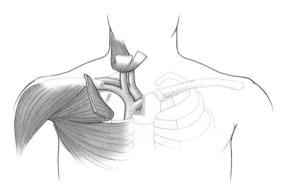

Fig. 2. Borders of the resection margin are shown. The medial one-third of the clavicle, the hemimanubrium, and the medial end of the first rib are removed. (*Reprinted from* Kachala S, D'Souza DM, Teixeira-Johnson L, et al. Surgical management of sternoclavicular joint infections. Ann Thorac Surg 2016;101:2155–60; with permission.)

the face of infection: (1) primary closure with or without muscle flap, (2) delayed primary closure with or without muscle flap, or (3) healing by secondary intention aided or not by vacuum dressing. The most common method of closure using a muscle flap is an ipsilateral pectoralis advancement flap based on the thoracoacromial artery. This artery arises from the subclavian artery, coming out under the lateral third of the clavicle. It is typically out of the area of debridement. If a larger flap is needed, the latissimus major muscle or rectus femoris muscle (if the internal mammary is intact) can be used.

Carlos and colleagues[46] reported the earliest experience using delayed primary closure (n = 1), primary closure (n = 3), and a single stage resection with ipsilateral pectoralis muscle flap (n = 4). Two patients died, including one from endocarditis 1 month after incision and drainage rather than SC joint resection, but the remaining patients' wounds healed without complication. Song and colleagues[41] reported their series of 7 patients in 2002. Six patients were treated initially with incision and drainage in conjunction with antibiotic therapy. Five of the 6 patients failed this therapy, requiring formal resection of the SCJ with partial manubrium resection and rib resection as indicated. The wounds were closed with an ipsilateral pectoralis advancement flap. The 6 patients treated with this approach had no wound complications and reported "normal" function at long-term follow-up (mean of 28 months). Burkhart and colleagues[40] reported 6 patients undergoing incision and debridement. Two patients had primary wound closure, 2 had delayed primary closure, and 2 were allowed to heal by secondary intention. An additional 20 patients underwent SJC resection. Of these 20 patients, 2 had primary closure, 6 healed by secondary intention, and 12 had delayed primary closure. Additionally, 11 of the joint resections had an ipsilateral pectoralis advancement flap done either at the initial procedure or at a later date. They reported only 1 wound-related complication that required the reopening of a closed wound owing to recurrent infection. Puri and colleagues[47] compared 10 patients undergoing a single-stage joint resection with ipsilateral pectoralis muscle flap closure with 10 patients undergoing joint resection and healing by secondary intention. The single-stage procedure resulted in significantly more wound complications consisting of hematoma, seroma, and wound dehiscence requiring surgical reexploration. The patients allowed to heal by secondary intention underwent wound care for a median of 12 weeks. Finally, the most recent and largest series to date was reported by Kachala and colleagues[43] in 2016. Forty patients treated surgically for SCJ infection over a 20-year period underwent either complete resection of the SCJ and then primary closure with ipsilateral pectoralis advancement flap or healing by secondary intention with negative pressure wound therapy. They reported no difference in outcome between these 2 methods of closure with regard to hospital duration of stay, antibiotic duration, wound complication rate (13% and 4%, respectively), and recurrence of infection (7% and 12%, respectively). Between these 2 groups, postclosure functional outcomes were reported as similar using a validated tool to access upper extremity dysfunction (QuickDASH Score) and both postoperative scores were within a range considered normal function.[48] In summary, the current literature suggests that multiple methods of closure can be successful in the treatment of SCJ infections and the chosen method should be personalized to the patient's risk factors and the extent of infection.

These authors propose the following suggestions when encountered with this disease process in a high-risk patient population.

1. A 1-week course of antibiotics, although it will not cure the joint infection, does not worsen the joint infection and often decreases the surrounding soft tissue swelling. This treatment will often make a single-stage procedure more likely and the overlying pectoralis major muscle a better candidate for soft tissue coverage.
2. Joint resection and closure by secondary intention requires approximately 3 months of wound care. Some patients do not have the personal resources, family support, or aid from the community to succeed with this plan, especially those patients suffering from substance abuse or mental health issues. Appropriate resources should be confirmed before leaving them with an open wound. In a select group of high-risk patients, chronic or intermittent antibiotics without resection may be a safer alternative therapy.

SUMMARY

Acute chest wall infections are uncommon and share similar risk factors for infection at other surgical sites. Smoking cessation has been shown to decrease the risk of SSI. Depending on the depth of infection and/or involvement of the organ space, adequate therapy usually involves a combination of antibiotics and drainage of the infected space. Early diagnosis and debridement of necrotizing soft tissue infections is essential to reduce the risk of mortality. SCJ infections often require surgical debridement with en bloc resection of the joint in addition to antibiotic therapy. Published reports suggest minimal long-term dysfunction despite en bloc joint resection. A standard approach to wound closure after resection has yet to be established. VAC is a valuable adjunct to standard therapy and can be used in all types of chest wall and pleural space infections.

REFERENCES

1. Mangram AJ, Horan TC, Pearson ML, et al. Guideline for Prevention of Surgical Site Infection, 1999. Centers for Disease Control and Prevention (CDC) Hospital Infection Control Practices Advisory Committee. Am J Infect Control 1999;27(2):97–132 [quiz: 133–4; discussion: 96].
2. Young P, Khadaroo R. Surgical site infections. Surg Clin North Am 2014;94:1245–64.
3. Alexander J, Solomkin JS, Edwards MJ. Updated recommendations for control of surgical site infections. Ann Surg 2011;253(6):1082–93.
4. Jensen JA, Goodson WH, Hopf HW, et al. Cigarette smoking decreases tissue oxygen. Arch Surg 1991; 126:1131–4.
5. Mason DS, Nowicki S, Grab ER, et al. Impact of smoking cessation before resection of lung cancer: a Society of Thoracic Surgeons General Thoracic Database Study. Ann Thorac Surg 2009;88:362–71.
6. Kozower BD, Sheng S, O'Brien SM, et al. STS database risk models: predictors of mortality and major morbidity for lung cancer resection. Ann Thorac Surg 2010;90(3):875–81; discussion 881–73.
7. Fernandez FG, Kosinski AS, Burfeind W, et al. The Society of Thoracic Surgeons Lung Cancer Resection

Risk Model: Higher Quality Data and Superior Outcomes. Ann Thorac Surg 2016;102(2):370–7.

8. Barrera R, Shi W, Amar D, et al. Smoking and timing of cessation: impact on pulmonary complications after thoracotomy. Chest 2005;127(6):1977–83.

9. Kozower BD, Sheng S, O'Brien SM, et al. STS database risk models: predictors of mortality and major morbidity for lung cancer resection. Ann Thorac Surg 2010;90(3):875–81 [discussion: 881–3].

10. Sziklavari Z, Ried M, Neu R, et al. Mini-open vacuum-assisted closure therapy with instillation for debilitated and septic patients with pleural empyema. Eur J Cardiothorac Surg 2015;48:e9–16.

11. Lindstrom D, Sadr Azodi O, Wladis A, et al. Effects of a perioperative smoking cessation intervention on postoperative complications: a randomized trial. Ann Surg 2008;248(5):739–45.

12. Møller AM, Villebro N, Pedersen T, et al. Effect of preoperative smoking intervention on postoperative complications: a randomised clinical trial. Lancet 2002;359(9301):114–7.

13. Thomsen T, Tønnesen H, Møller AM. Effect of preoperative smoking cessation interventions on postoperative complications and smoking cessation. Br J Surg 2009;96:451–61.

14. Fleischmann WS, Bombelli W, Kinzl M. Vacuum sealing as treatment of soft tissue damage in open fractures. Unfallchirurg 1993;96:488–92.

15. Müllner T, Mrkonjic L, Kwasny O, et al. The use of negative pressure to promote the healing of tissue defects: a clinical trial using the vacuum sealing technique. Br J Plast Surg 1997;50:194–9.

16. O'Connor J, Kells A, Henry S, et al. Vacuum-assisted closure for the treatment of complex chest wounds. Ann Thorac Surg 2005;79:1196–200.

17. Varker K, Ng T. Management of empyema cavity with the vacuum-assisted closure device. Ann Thorac Surg 2006;81:723–5.

18. Philbeck TE Jr, Whittington KT, Millsap MH, et al. The clinical and cost effectiveness of externally applied negative pressure wound therapy in the treatment of wounds in home healthcare Medicare patients. Ostomy Wound Manage 1999;45(11):41–50.

19. Morykwas MJ, Argenta LC, Shelton-Brown EI, et al. Vacuum-assisted closure: a new method for wound control and treatment: animal studies and basic foundation. Ann Plast Surg 1997;38:553–62.

20. Hunter JE, Teot L, Horch R. Evidenced-based medicine: vacuum-assisted closure in wound care management. Int Wound J 2007;4:256–69.

21. Welvaart WN, Oosterhuis JW, Paul MA. Negative pressure dressing for radiation-associated wound dehiscence after posterolateral thoracotomy. Interact Cardiovasc Thorac Surg 2009;8:558–60.

22. Davis JS, Kourliouros A, Deshpande R, et al. Novel technique for avoidance of pressure competition between a negative pressure wound therapy device and chest drains in the management of deep sternal wound infections. Interact Cardiovasc Thorac Surg 2015;20(2):270–2.

23. Begum S, Papagiannopoulos K. The use of vacuum-assisted wound closure therapy in thoracic operations. Ann Thorac Surg 2012;94:1835–40.

24. Palmen M, van Breugel HN, Geskes GG, et al. Open window thoracostomy treatment of empyema is accelerated by vacuum-assisted closure. Ann Thorac Surg 2009;88:1131–7.

25. Haghshenasskashani A, Rahnavardi M, Yan TD, et al. Intrathoracic application of a vacuum-assisted closure device in managing pleural space infection after lung resection: is it an option? Interact Cardiovasc Thorac Surg 2011;13(2):168–74.

26. Sziklavari Z, Ried M, Neu R, et al. Mini-open vacuum-assisted closure therapy with instillation for debilitated and septic patients with pleural empyema. Eur J Cardiothorac Surg 2015;48(2):e9–16.

27. Hofmann HS, Neu R, Potzger T, et al. Minimally invasive vacuum-assisted closure therapy with instillation (Mini-VAC-Instill) for pleural empyema. Surg Innov 2015;22(3):235–9.

28. Saadi A, Perentes JY, Gonzalez M, et al. Vacuum-assisted closure device: a useful tool in the management of severe intrathoracic infections. Ann Thorac Surg 2011;91:1582–90.

29. Groetzner J, Holzer M, Stockhausen D, et al. Intrathoracic application of vacuum wound therapy following thoracic surgery. Thorac Cardiovasc Surg 2009;57:417–20.

30. Losanoff JE, Richman BW, Jones JW. Necrotizing soft tissue infection of the chest wall. Ann Thorac Surg 2002;73:304–6.

31. Goh T, Goh LG, Ang CH, et al. Early diagnosis of necrotizing fasciitis. Br J Surg 2014;101(1):e119–125.

32. Morgan M. Diagnosis and management of necrotising fasciitis: a multiparametric approach. J Hosp Infect 2010;75:249–57.

33. Sarani B, Strong M, Pascual J, et al. Necrotizing fasciitis: current concepts and review of the literature. J Am Coll Surg 2009;208(2):279–88.

34. Jallali NW, Butter S, Butler PE. Hyperbaric oxygen therapy. Am J Surg 2005;189:462–6.

35. Roje Z, Roje Z, Matić D, et al. Necrotizing fasciitis: literature review of contemporary strategies for diagnosing and management with three case reports: torso, abdominal wall, upper and lower limbs. World J Emerg Surg 2011;4(46):1–17.

36. Ross J, Shamsuddin H. Sternoclavicular septic arthritis: review of 180 cases. Medicine 2004;83(3):139–48.

37. Renfree K, Wright T. Anatomy and biomechanics of the acromioclavicular and sternoclavicular joints. Clin Sports Med 2003;22:219–37.

38. Acus RB, Bell RH, Fisher DL. Proximal clavicle excision: an analysis of results. J Shoulder Elbow Surg 1995;4:182–7.

39. Song HK, Guy TS, Kaiser LR, et al. Current presentation and optimal surgical management of sternoclavicular joint infections. Ann Thorac Surg 2002; 73(2):427–31.

40. Burkhart H, Deschamps C, Allen MS, et al. Surgical management of sternoclavicular joint infections. J Thorac Cardiovasc Surg 2003;125:945–9.

41. Song HK, Guy TS, Kaiser LR, et al. Current presentation and optimal surgical management of sternoclavicular joint infections. Ann Thorac Surg 2002;73: 427–31.

42. Sorensen L, Karlsmark T, Gottrup F. Abstinence from smoking reduces incisional wound infection: a randomized controlled trial. Ann Surg 2003; 238(1):1–5.

43. Kachala SS, D'Souza DM, Teixeira-Johnson L, et al. Surgical management of sternoclavicular joint infections. Ann Thorac Surg 2016;101:2155–60.

44. Ross J, Shamsuddin H. Sternoclavicular septic arthritis: review of 180 cases. Medicine 2004;83:139–48.

45. Hofmann H, Schemm R, Grosser C, et al. Vacuum-assisted closure of pleural empyema without classic open-window thoracostomy. Ann Thorac Surg 2012; 93:1741–2.

46. Carlos G, Kesler KA, Coleman JJ, et al. Aggressive surgical management of sternoclavicular joint infections. J Thorac Cardiovasc Surg 1997;113:242–7.

47. Puri V, Meyers BF, Kreisel D, et al. Sternoclavicular joint infection: a comparison of two surgical approaches. Ann Thorac Surg 2011;91(1):257–61.

48. Kachala SS, D'Souza DM, Teixeira-Johnson L, et al. Surgical management of sternoclavicular joint infections. Ann Thorac Surg 2016;101(6):2155–60.

Chronic Infections of the Chest Wall

Edward J. Bergeron, MD*, Robert A. Meguid, MD, MPH, John D. Mitchell, MD

KEYWORDS

- Infection • Chest wall • Osteomyelitis • Sternoclavicular joint • Tuberculosis • Granuloma

KEY POINTS

- Chronic chest wall infections may occur in soft tissue, cartilage, and bone. Infectious pathogens may be bacterial, fungal, or parasitic.
- They may present as a discrete mass and can initially be mistaken for a neoplasm, a superficial infection, or a draining sinus.
- Effective management of chronic chest wall infections ranges from antibiotic administration to wide surgical resection of all devitalized tissue and subsequent coverage with well-vascularized soft tissue.
- Secondary sternal osteomyelitis is associated with complications of median sternotomy.
- Infectious seeding of the sternoclavicular joint is typically via hematogenous route.

INTRODUCTION

Chronic chest wall infections are rare, and those necessitating surgical consultation are even more uncommon. They result from direct inoculation of the chest wall or from contiguous or hematogenous spread from infected tissue, or from previous chest wall trauma or instrumentation. Chronic chest wall infections may occur in soft tissue, cartilage, and bone. Infectious pathogens may be bacterial, fungal, or parasitic. The diagnosis of chronic chest wall infections is difficult because of subtle, nonspecific signs, symptoms, and presentations, and because of their clinical rarity. They may present as localized chest wall pain, a discrete mass initially mistaken for neoplasm, a superficial infection, or a draining sinus. Effective management of chest wall infections ranges from antimicrobial administration to wide surgical resection of all devitalized tissue and subsequent coverage with well-vascularized soft tissue. Treatment depends on the type, magnitude, and location of the

infection. Prompt timing in the diagnosis and treatment is important to minimize associated morbidities. This article presents a systematic review of chronic chest wall infections, and their associated work-up and management.

Chronic chest wall infections are typically nonnecrotizing and associated with lower morbidity than their more acute and necrotizing counterparts. They may often respond to nonsurgical management, but knowledge of their presentation and management is important to thoracic surgeons. Because of the chronic nature of the infection and subsequent prolonged inflammation, wound healing associated with chronic chest wall infections may result in differing degrees of fibrosis, aiding in the structural integrity of the chest wall if surgical therapy is needed. This is in contrast to their acute necrotizing infection counterparts, where the rapid onset of the infection does not allow for underlying fibrosis. If radical surgical debridement is required for chronic chest wall infection management, blood supply and

Disclosures: The authors have no disclosures.
Division of Cardiothoracic Surgery, Department of Surgery, University of Colorado, Anschutz Medical Campus, 12631 East 17th Avenue, C-310, Aurora, CO 80045, USA
* Corresponding author.
E-mail address: Edward.Bergeron@ucdenver.edu

Thorac Surg Clin 27 (2017) 87–97
http://dx.doi.org/10.1016/j.thorsurg.2017.01.002
1547-4127/17/© 2017 Elsevier Inc. All rights reserved.

resulting wound healing can be compromised as a result of the fibrosis. Common and rare chronic chest wall infections are discussed next.

CARTILAGE AND BONE INFECTIONS
Costochondral Infection

Infections of the costal cartilage, spanning the boney rib to the sternum, occur because of inoculation of the tissue by bacteria, or less commonly fungi. Most costochondral infections result from surgical intervention. However, costochondral infections may occur subsequent to penetrating trauma or via hematogenous spread from other sources of infection within the body. Most iatrogenic costochondral infections follow median sternotomy for cardiac surgery. In addition, thoracotomy and tube thoracostomy have been identified as inciting surgical trauma resulting in costochondral infections. Infection of the xiphoid cartilage may result in spread of infection bilaterally to the chest wall and costal cartilages.

Costochondral infections typically present as progressive discomfort, or pain of the anterior chest wall over time accompanied by localized tenderness on palpation, low-grade fever, leukocytosis, overlying erythema, and rarely, a draining sinus. In situations where the patient has undergone prior surgery or trauma to the area, nonunion of the involved ribs may result in instability beyond the expected time required for routine surgical healing. Wounds healing via secondary intention may result in a narrow, granulating wound with the underlying infected cartilage persistently exposed. As the overlying soft tissue and skin granulates with time, the chronically infected underlying cartilage serves as a nidus for a draining sinus.

Diagnosis of costochondral infection is made through a combination of clinical suspicion caused by a compelling history, prolonged duration of symptoms, physical examination, and imaging to guide local therapy. On interview with the patient, one can often elicit a history of discreet chest wall trauma, such as surgery. This is often followed by a prodromal period of chest wall pain on exertion, progressing to pain with minimal activity and respiration. Accompanying fevers, if any, are often low grade. Physical examination demonstrates tenderness over the chest wall adjacent to the nearby infection. Laboratory work-up may be notable for mildly elevated leukocytosis and elevated erythrocyte sedimentation rate and C-reactive protein. MRI is the imaging modality of choice because it may demonstrate tissue edema not well visualized on computed tomography (CT) scan.

Treatment of costochondral infection is a combination of the use of targeted antimicrobials and surgical resection of the infected connective tissue. Given the difficulty in identification of causative pathogens of most costochondral infections, broad-spectrum antibiotics targeted at gram-positive bacteria (eg, Staphylococcus aureus and Staphylococcus epidermidis) should be instituted. Surgery is indicated when symptoms persist, or findings on physical examination or radiographic imaging are compelling of infection refractory to antibiotics alone. Surgical treatment involves resection of the infected cartilage and surrounding infected soft tissue. Because the seventh through tenth costal cartilages are contiguous, infection involving any part of this costal cartilage typically requires resection of the entire costal arch unilaterally to achieve control. Samples of infected tissue should be sent for Gram stain and culture at the time of debridement.

Management of chest wall defects resulting from wide resection of costochondral infection depends on the extent of the defect. In the authors' experience, most defects resulting from treatment of costochondral infections are not full thickness with most of the skin, intercostal muscle, and perichondrium preserved. The resulting defects are managed with local soft tissue transposition, wet-to-dry dressings, or negative-pressure dressings with ongoing antibiotic administration.

Tubercular abscesses

Classically, abscesses are thought to occur in acute spectrum of infections. Additionally, extrapulmonary tubercular infections account for a minority of tuberculosis infections. Tuberculosis infections of the chest wall account for only 10% of extrapulmonary tuberculosis infections and are typically chronic infections.[1] However, a resurgence of tuberculosis in recent decades, largely as a result of proliferation of immunosuppressive conditions combined with immigration of people from developing nations to North America, has resulted in this being a more common entity of chronic chest wall infections.[2]

Tubercular abscesses of the chest wall have a strong predilection to the sternal margins. However, they may additionally involve ribs, costochondral junctions, costovertebral joints, and the vertebrae. Predilection to the sternal margin has been suggested to be the result from internal mammary lymph node infections secondary to primary pulmonary involvement. The infected lymph nodes then caseate, erode through the chest wall, and result in visible "swelling." The subpleural collections of this caseating material from the infected, necrosed lymph nodes are known as "cold abscesses." Bone erosion by tuberculosis results from pressure necrosis caused by the granulation tissue, or contiguous spread resulting in bone infection.

Multidrug systemic therapy is the mainstay for tuberculosis infections. However, treatment of cold abscesses includes the addition of aggressive surgical debridement and wide excision of the bone and infected soft tissue to prevent recurrence.[1,3] Muscle flap reconstruction of the sternum typically follows.

Osteomyelitis of the Chest Wall

Primary chest wall osteomyelitis is most frequently associated with illicit intravenous drug abuse or traumatic inoculation. Secondary sternal osteomyelitis is associated with complications of cardiothoracic surgery. Patients typically present with localized chest wall pain, with or without low-grade fever. On physical examination, they may have localized chest wall tenderness, erythema, swollen soft tissue, and occasionally, sinus tract

formation overlying the infected bone (**Fig. 1**A). Laboratory studies may demonstrate mild leukocytosis, or no elevation in white blood cell count at all, and elevated erythrocyte sedimentation rate and C-reactive protein.

Osteomyelitis and associated changes to tissue surrounding the infected bone are visualized on plain radiograph, ultrasonography, CT scan, MRI, or nuclear medicine bone scan. Imaging from CT scan and noncontrast MRI are most useful for guiding treatment and planning surgery. Imaging may reveal fluid collections, edema or air surrounding the infected bone, and changes to the bone consistent with osteomyelitis (**Fig. 1**B, C).

Ideally, bone biopsies and concomitant blood cultures should be obtained before institution of antimicrobial therapy. Bone biopsies are achieved via a needle biopsy or an open surgical biopsy. However, negative cultures should not supersede clinical suspicion of infection. A recent review of image-guided percutaneous biopsies for osteomyelitis demonstrated a low probability of identifying specific microbes. Less than 10% of

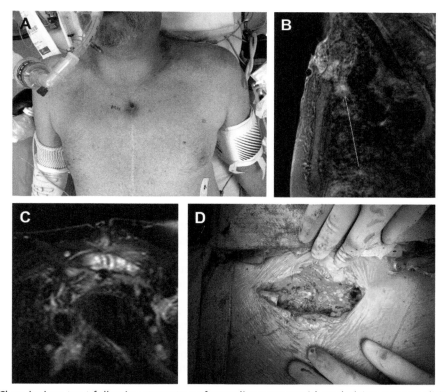

Fig. 1. (A) Chronic sinus tract following sternotomy for cardiac surgery with underlying osteomyelitis of the manubrium and clavicular heads. (B) Sagital T1-weighted image from MRI demonstrating low signal with enhancement of the manubrium and abnormal enhancement of T1 hypointensity extending posterior to the sternum into the anterior mediastinum at the level of the sternomanubrial articulation (arrow). (C) Axial T2-weighted MRI demonstrating high enhancement of manubrium. (D) Complete surgical excision of involved bone and the overlying soft tissue was performed. (Courtesy of Robert Meguid, MD, MPH, Aurora, CO.)

biopsies resulted in additional information for the identification of the pathologic microorganism present or changed treatment regimens.[4] The successful treatment of chronic osteomyelitis entails administration of targeted antimicrobials, extensive surgical debridement of infected and devascularized tissue, followed with myocutaneous reconstruction (**Fig. 1**D). Examples of common chest wall osteomyelitis chronic infections are discussed next.

Osteomyelitis of the Sternum

Although primary sternal osteomyelitis is associated with intravenous drug abuse, secondary sternal osteomyelitis occurs in 1% to 3% of patients following sternotomy, usually for cardiac surgery. The most significant risk factor for secondary sternal osteomyelitis is reoperation for excessive postoperative bleeding following cardiac surgery. Other risk factors for postoperative sternal infections include diabetes mellitus, low cardiac output, and the use of bilateral internal mammary artery grafts during coronary artery bypass and grafting.[5]

Joint effusions at the sternomanubrial joint may be present. In the setting of prior sternotomy, patients may have an unstable sternum with serosanguineous drainage. Findings on imaging that may raise suspicion of an indolent, chronic sternal osteomyelitis include malunion of the sternotomy, and broken or avulsed sternal wires or closure devices.[6] Debridement of infected of nonvascular sternal tissue followed with bilateral pectoralis muscle flap advancement is the most common method for management and soft tissue coverage of poststernotomy osteomyelitis, when available.[7]

Osteomyelitis of the Ribs

Osteomyelitis of the ribs is less commonly encountered than that of the sternum. It is usually diagnosed because of local pain, tenderness, and inflammation with or without the presence of a chronic, persistent draining sinus tract. Osteomyelitis of the ribs is typically caused by the traumatic inoculation by *S aureus* either secondary to trauma or surgery. On imaging, any intrapleural nidus of infection perpetuating a persistent draining sinus should be identified (**Fig. 2**). In the setting of osteomyelitis of the ribs, we have encountered parenchyma-pleural fistulas and foreign material, such as nonabsorbable braided sutures resulting in chronic infection. Excision of all infected bone, treatment of the cause for the underlying fistula, and local soft tissue coverage, followed by prolonged antibiotic administration, is typically required for eradication of osteomyelitis of the ribs.

Osteomyelitis of the Sternoclavicular Joint

The sternoclavicular joint consists of the lateral notch of the manubrium, the medial inferior head of the clavicle, and the costocartilage of the first rib. It is a gliding synovial joint and has minimal soft tissue coverage. Infections of the sternoclavicular joint only represent 2% of pyogenic arthritis. However, 20% of sternoclavicular infected patients may develop a sternoclavicular joint–related abscess as a result of the joint capsule's inability to distend.[8] Intravenous drug use, immunosuppression including diabetes and long-term steroid use, chronic hemodialysis, subclavian venous catheters, and local trauma including surgery are all predisposing factors for sternoclavicular joint infections.[9] Tracheostomy in patients with short necks, or created low down on the manubrium, are predisposed to development of osteomyelitis of the manubrium and sternoclavicular joint (**Fig. 3**A). Women having undergone breast irradiation for breast cancer may also have a late presentation of sternoclavicular joint septic arthritis decades following their radiation treatments.[10]

Infectious seeding of the sternoclavicular joint is typically via the hematogenous route. However, direct contiguous spread of infection may also result in a septic sternoclavicular joint. *S aureus* is the predominant organism present in the general population. *Pseudomonas aeruginosa* historically is reported as being more typical in intravenous drug users.[11] However, recent evidence suggests *S aureus* is still the major pathogen for the general population and intravenous drug abusers.[12] The thoracic surgeon plays a central role in the management of the sternoclavicular joint infection because of its proximity to the pleural space, mediastinum, and brachiocephalic structures.

Most (95%) pyogenic sternoclavicular joint infections are unilateral. Occurrence on the right side is slightly greater than the left. Patient presentation includes sternoclavicular joint pain with or without shoulder pain and 65% may have associated fever. Physical findings include focal tenderness with joint swelling, skin erythema, and associated induration depending on extent of the infection.[12]

Imaging of sternoclavicular joint infections can be troublesome. Plain radiograph and ultrasound are unreliable in the early phase of this prolonged infection. Ultrasound is useful for joint effusions, enlargement of the joint synovium, and associated soft tissue collections.[13] CT scan is the preferred diagnostic imaging to help the thoracic surgeon to determine the spatial relationship of the sternoclavicular joint infection to the remaining chest

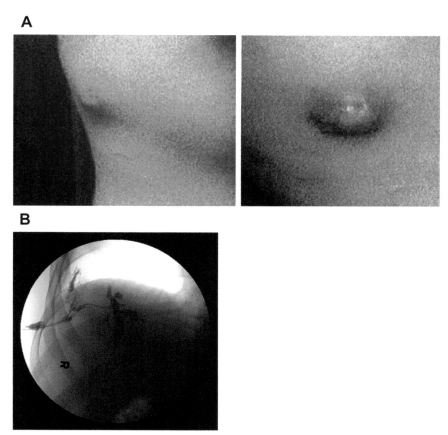

Fig. 2. (*A*) Chronic sinus tract from underlying rib osteomyelitis following prolonged tube thoracostomy presenting 9 years after right thoracoscopic pleurodesis for spontaneous pneumothorax, followed by two subsequent thoracotomies and exploration and decortication for recurrent hematoma and empyema in the right chest of a patient with hemophilia. (*B*) Sinogram of sinus tract. This patient was treated surgically with excision of the underlying infected rib and debridement of the associated overlying soft tissue with local tissue advancement flap coverage and a prolonged course of culture-directed antimicrobials. (*Courtesy of* Robert Meguid, MD, MPH, Aurora, CO.)

wall, pleural space, and vessels. CT scan also images sternoclavicular joint-related bone erosion and sclerosis in patients presenting subacutely, and potentially new bone formation associated with chronic infections. However, bone scan and MRI may better demonstrate signs of osteomyelitis (see **Fig. 3**). Patients who have a sternoclavicular joint infection associated with hematogenous seeding, as opposed to contiguous spread, should undergo echocardiogram to determine if valve vegetations are the cause of bloodstream inoculation with the offending bacteria.

The management of pyogenic septic arthritis depends on the extent of the infection. Sternoclavicular joint infections without extracapsular fluid collections or bony destruction are managed medically with administration of broad-spectrum antibiotics and removal of potential seeding sources (ie, central venous catheters).[12] Incision and drainage may suffice for those joints with limited infection or when a histopathologic specimen is needed for diagnosis guidance of antibiotic therapy. However, simple incision and drainage is unlikely to resolve the infection.[9,14] Surgical debridement is typically required for adequate treatment. Wide *en bloc* resection of the joint and involved soft tissue or piecemeal debridement of all nonviable tissue and involved structures is commonly required when periarticular fluid, abscess, bone destruction, or persistent infection have developed despite an extended course of antibiotic administration.

Resection of an infected sternoclavicular joint proceeds as follows: (1) a hockey-stick incision is made extending laterally over the medial half of the clavicle, and inferiorly down the manubrium to the first intercostal space to allow access to the sternoclavicular joint; (2) viable pectoralis and

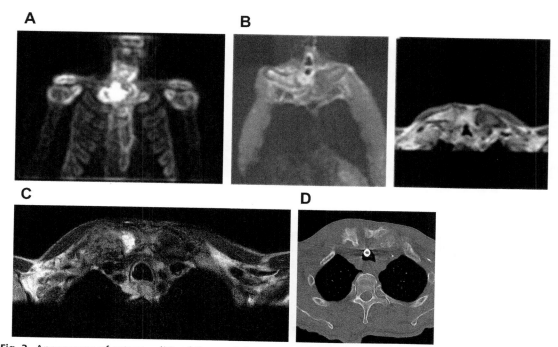

Fig. 3. Appearance of osteomyelitis of the medial right clavicle and adjacent manubrium, with inflammation of surrounding tissue, in a 70-year-old man with a long in-dwelling tracheostomy appliance. (*A*) Edge-enhanced nuclear medicine scan. (*B*) T1-weighted postcontrast MRI demonstrating confluent T1 hypointense enhancing signal involving the medial third of the right clavicle and an effusion within the right sternoclavicular joint with associated prominent capsular and synovial enhancement. Note the differential enhancement of the right medial clavicular head versus the left. (*C*) T2-weighted precontrast MRI demonstrating T2 hyperintense, enhancing signal within the bone marrow of the right clavicular head. (*D*) Axial CT scan demonstrating sclerosis of the bone but lack of clear indications of osteomyelitis. This patient underwent resection of the medial third of the right clavicle and adjacent manubrium, and debridement of the adjacent soft tissue, with delayed secondary closure using negative-pressure wound therapy. Concurrently, he was treated with a prolonged course of culture-directed antibiotics.

sternocleidomastoid muscle fibers are resected away from areas of phlegmon and all involved tissue is widely debrided; (3) the clavicle lateral to the area of osteomyelitis is circumferentially exposed, with care to protect the underlying subclavian vein and artery; (4) the clavicle is divided 2-cm lateral to the inflammatory mass using an oscillating saw and the clavicular head is resected; and (5) the remaining involved soft tissue, sternoclavicular joint, and adjacent manubrium is debrided with rongeurs and/or curettes. Soft tissue and bone is sent for microbiologic assessment and culture. Limiting resection to half of the manubrium is important to maintain chest wall stability. The costal cartilage and medial portion of the first rib are divided with rib shears if involved, although this is rare.[9,14]

Serial debridement of sternoclavicular infections is occasionally required to ensure all devitalized and infected material is removed. A temporary negative-pressure dressing or wet-to-dry dressings using Dakin solution is useful between episodes of debridement. The exposed divided clavicle and manubrium are covered with locally advanced soft tissue, including the strap muscles of the neck or the superior part of the pectoralis major muscle, and allowed to heal by secondary intention. Most resulting wounds respond well to negative-pressure dressings. Occasionally the resulting defect is large and requires more complex soft tissue coverage for closure. An ipsilateral pectoralis muscle advancement flap is well situated to cover the defect. Simultaneously, long-term antimicrobials are administered. Despite the aggressive nature of debridement of infected sternoclavicular joints, postoperative shoulder function is usually well preserved, and most patients report long-term normal upper extremity performance.

In a series of 26 patients with sternoclavicular joint infections, patients reported pain as the most common symptom followed by swelling over the infected sternoclavicular joint.[14] Five of the patients had a trauma history, and half of the patients reported ongoing or recent infections. Patients were treated with antibiotics for a median of 42 days following surgical drainage or debridement. Four patients had undergone previous incision and drainage, and wound cultures were positive in most patients. Unilateral debridement was the treatment most commonly used, allowing for the eventual use of an ipsilateral pectoralis muscle flap for coverage and closure.

Atypical infections of the sternoclavicular joints may also occur. Extraspinal tubercular arthritis may occur at the sternoclavicular joint.[15] Tubercular infections of the sternoclavicular joint may have characteristic radiologic findings including an inflammatory mass, abscess wall calcification, and absence of new bone formation. Compression of the subclavian vessels by this inflammatory mass may also be found. Microbiologic and histologic studies are important to make a definitive diagnosis, but can be delayed because of the slow-growing nature of many of these atypical organisms. Treatment is as described for more commonly occurring sternoclavicular joint infections, with use of prolonged chemotherapy targeted to tuberculosis.

Brucella sternoclavicular arthritis is rare, but has been reported.[16] *Brucella* are gram-negative, facultative anaerobes found in domesticated animals. It is endemic in parts of Central America, the Mediterranean, Middle East, and Asia. Human infections may result from consumption of infected meat and milk consumption. Musculoskeletal involvement is the common human manifestation. The infection is systemic. Sternoclavicular joint infection occurs in the minority of cases (2%–5%).[17] Definitive diagnosis requires microbiologic organism confirmation, or antibody serology. Treatment is 6 to 12 weeks of streptomycin and doxycycline or tetracycline to eradicate the organism from the bone. Surgical debridement is seldom necessary for *Brucella* sternoclavicular infections.

CHRONIC INFECTIONS OF THE CHEST WALL SOFT TISSUES
Empyema Necessitans

Empyema necessitans results from an undrained, underlying pleural infection. This infection is commonly polymicrobial and is the direct extension of an untreated, chronic empyema that extends through the chest wall into the superficial tissue of the chest. Physical examination and axial radiographic imaging of the chest (eg, chest CT imaging) elucidate the diagnosis (**Fig. 4**). Definitive treatment includes antibiotic administration, surgical drainage of the empyema, and debridement of devitalized tissue from the site of necessitation through the chest wall. Spontaneous drainage of the empyema necessitans is inadequate treatment.

Chest Wall Actinomycosis

Actinomycosis of the chest wall is a rare thoracic infection.[18] It is a chronic disease characterized by chronic granulomas or abscesses, which eventually progress to draining sinuses discharging bacterial microcolonies with the appearance of "sulfur granules." *Actinomyces* is a gram-positive anaerobic bacteria commonly found in healthy

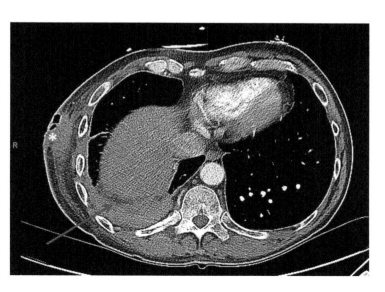

Fig. 4. CT scan of empyema necessitans. A right loculated empyema (*arrow*) with direct communication of the chest wall (*asterisk*) consistent with empyema necessitans.

human and animal oral flora. There are three major infectious regions of actinomycosis: (1) cervicofacial (most common, 65%), (2) abdominal (20%), and (3) thoracic (15%).

The thoracic form usually results from aspiration by a patient with poor oral hygiene. Thoracic *Actinomyces* infection subsequently develops within the lung parenchyma and over time, can progress through the pleura, necessitating out of the chest wall. Thoracic actinomycosis may be complicated by hemoptysis, systemic spread, a chronic draining sinus, or empyema.[19]

Hematogenous spread of actinomycosis is rare, but when occurs typically has a persistent thoracic origin. This disseminated form of the disease may result in distant abscesses, including the brain. Localized chest wall infections caused by *Actinomyces*, without pulmonary involvement, are rare and are often misidentified as locally advanced primary chest wall tumors.

Actinomycotic chest wall infections are diagnosed by isolating *Actinomyces* in culture. However, the organism is difficult to grow in culture medium and subsequently false-negative cultures may result. A surgical biopsy is commonly necessary to provide tissue for histopathologic confirmation of the presence of the pathognomonic grainy microcolonies, or "sulfur granules." Actinomycosis of the chest wall is treated with incision, drainage, and debridement of the affected areas and long-term penicillin therapy.[20]

Fungal Infections

Fungal infections of the chest wall may occur and are commonly a result of chronic infection.

Aspergillus chest wall infections may result from primary direct infection or from a disseminated infection. These typically present as an indurated plaque progressing to a necrotic ulcer of the skin. On histologic evaluation, *Aspergillus* chest wall infections are characterized by branching septate hyphae.

Phycomyces histologically appear as broad-based nonseptate hyphae. Other organisms associated with chronic chest wall infections include *Mucor* or *Rhizopus* species. The surgical component of treatment requires debridement until a margin of normal-appearing, granuloma-free tissue on frozen pathologic examination is achieved. Debridement is accompanied by concurrent and prolonged antifungal chemotherapy.

Chronic Parasitic Infections

Parasitic infections may involve the chest wall. Although these are rarely encountered in North America, they may be encountered in patients living in, or whom have traveled from, endemic areas. A few different parasites are notable for chest wall involvement, and are discussed next.

Leishmaniasis, caused by the protozoan parasite *Leishmania*, is transmitted by the bite of the Phlebotomine sand fly. It is endemic in parts of the Arabian Peninsula, Asia, Africa, South America, Central America, and southern Europe. Infection can manifest as a lingering cutaneous ulcer occurring weeks to months after the inoculating bite occurred. Diagnosis is based on clinical history, including travel exposure, and on physical examination. It can be treated with fluconazole, miltefosine, or pentamidine. Specific medical treatment depends on the species of *Leishmania* acquired, the type of infection, and the location where the disease was acquired. Surgery is typically reserved for cosmetic treatment of cutaneous lesions.[21]

Infection of soft tissue by parasitic larvae of myiatic flies can involve the chest wall. Myiasis is parasitic infestation of the living flesh. An example of this is by the *Cordylobia anthropophaga* (the tumbu fly or mango fly) species of the myiatic blow fly endemic to central and east Africa.[22] Diagnosis is based on clinical history, including travel exposure, and on physical examination. Treatment of this dramatic infection is elimination of the parasitic larvae by incision and debridement or extraction, with subsequent treatment with antiparasitic agents, such as ivermectin.[23]

Echinococcosis, or hydatid cyst formation by the larvae of the *Echinococcus* species of tapeworms, may occur in ribs. *Echinococcus* species are endemic in some areas of Africa, South America, and Asia. Although typically infesting the liver and lungs, bone involvement may rarely occur. Rib involvement accounts for 8% of bone hydatidosis.[24] The eggs of the *Echinococcus* species are ingested by humans as an accidental host. These eggs penetrate the small bowel wall, and disseminate hematogenously, typically to the liver and lungs but rarely to the chest wall. The eggs release embryos, which grow into cysts. These cysts typically grow 5 to 10 cm in size per year, and can survive in hosts for many years. Within cysts develop daughter cysts and protoscolices. Multiloculated pleural swelling is present and the disease can progress to destruction of cancellous bone and spread to the vertebral bodies.

Diagnosis of echinococcosis is based on clinical history, including travel exposure, and on physical examination. Imaging modalities to visualize the hydatid cysts include ultrasound, CT, and MRI, demonstrating presence of the fluid-filled cyst. Confirmation of diagnosis is achieved with serologic testing including enzyme-linked immunosorbent assay and indirect hemagglutination assay. Needle biopsy of the cyst may result in dissemination of the daughter cysts and protoscolices and is therefore contraindicated. Treatment is *en bloc* surgical resection of cystic lesions with negative margins, and sterilization of other sites of hydatidosis, such as the liver or lungs, either surgically or chemically. Rupture of the cysts during diagnosis or surgery may result in dissemination of the disease. Pretreatment and posttreatment chemotherapy is performed with albendazole or mebendazole, continued for 1 to 6 months after surgery.[25]

MANAGEMENT OF SURGICAL WOUNDS RESULTING FROM CHRONIC CHEST WALL INFECTIONS
Negative-Pressure Wound Therapy

The wide adoption of negative-pressure wound therapy, or vacuum-assisted closure technology, to complex wounds and more specifically chest wounds has proven effective.[26] These negative-pressure dressings accelerate wound healing and ultimately wound closure by continuously providing a wound bed environment with increased blood flow, drainage of excess fluid, and resulting decrease is tissue edema, while removing bacteria. The degree and schedule of subatmospheric pressure is varied depending on the device.[27] They have a particularly useful application for the treatment of chronic chest wall infections.

Negative-pressure wound therapy provided by these devices has been shown to alter wound bed cell cytoskeleton and trigger intracellular cascades increasing cell division, formation of granulation tissue, and ultimately promote wound healing.[28] The authors use this technique for small wounds with exposed soft tissue only, which do not enter the pleural space. We occasionally use negative-pressure wound therapy to stabilize and temporize an open sternum after serial debridements for sternal wound infections (**Fig. 5**). In the latter, we find the negative-pressure wound dressing promotes granulation tissue formation providing a bed for subsequent reconstruction with soft tissue flaps.

The wide and ever increasing availability of negative-pressure wound dressings combined with their few contraindications, low rate of complications, and relative portability have made them a mainstay of modern wound care. They are routinely managed in the outpatient setting, and ideal for subacute and chronic wounds. This outpatient management allows the patient to resume activities of daily living and for the elective

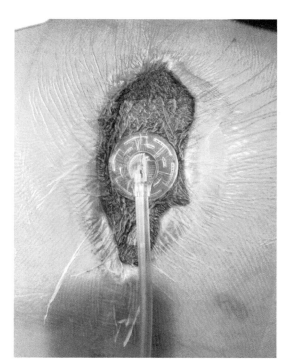

Fig. 5. An example of negative-pressure wound therapy after sternal dehiscence and development of osteomyelitis following cardiac surgery via median sternotomy. This modality is commonly used in the modern management of chest wall infections. (*Courtesy of* Ashok Babu, MD, Nashville, TN.)

scheduling of any subsequent surgical reconstruction. Negative-pressure wound dressing use in the chest has been shown to lessen inpatient hospital stays, decrease the number of required operative debridements, decreased rates of subsequent wound infection, and increase rates of primary wound closure.[29] Negative-pressure wound dressing application to thoracotomy incisions, including intrapleural application, and even in direct contact with the heart has proven safe.[30] The wide range and success of negative pressure wound dressing makes it an increasingly used tool in contemporary chest wall wound management.

Chest Wall Reconstruction

Large and varying-thickness soft tissue defects in the chest wall may result from surgical debridement of chronic chest wall infections. Resulting defects can pose challenges to wound reconstruction, closure, and management. This soft tissue coverage is difficult, not only because of the large size of some defects requiring repair, but because of the infectious involvement of the adjacent chest wall muscles, which are commonly used for tissue flaps in the more traditional chest wall reconstructions.

We strive to cover large and full-thickness chest wall defects resulting from treatment of infections with autologous tissue, minimizing foreign material that may themselves become nidus for infections. Although in depth review of chest wall reconstruction is beyond the scope of this article, soft tissue reconstruction can be performed using a combination of myocutaneous, muscle, and omental flaps; skin grafts; and free bone grafts. Muscles, such as the latissimus dorsi and serratus anterior, are used to cover exposed lung and mediastinal structures, as is omentum brought up into the chest through the diaphragm. Autologous ribs from a sterile, contralateral site are used as a free graft for large defects, in lieu of metallic prosthetics. We prefer to use pectoralis major advancement and rotational flaps for anterior defects, with bilateral pectoralis major advancement flaps covering and stabilizing sternal defects. For lateral and posterior defects, the latissimus dorsi and serratus anterior muscles are usually reasonably large and mobile to provide coverage. These muscle flaps can then accept skin grafts when necessary.

The use of prosthetic mesh for structural integrity is usually contraindicated because of the infectious risk. Thus, cadaveric and other biologic matrices have become an attractive option for skeletal reconstruction, even though they lack the long-term mechanics of their prosthetic counterparts. Delayed reconstruction with pure synthetic prosthetics, such as titanium, Gore-Tex (W. L. Gore & Associates, Inc, Newark, DE), or polypropylene mesh (Marlex, Chevron Phillips Chemical Company LLC, The Woodlands, TX), is possible once the infection has been convincingly cleared, but this is an exceedingly rare circumstance for chronic chest wall infections in our practice.

SUMMARY

Chronic chest wall infections involve a spectrum of presentations from extensive cellulitis to draining sinuses to discrete masses. Causes are broad, but include direct chest wall trauma, chest wall inoculation from systemic infection, and surgical intervention of the chest wall. Outcomes are affected by the rapidity of diagnosis and onset of definitive treatment, the causative organism, extent of the infection, and degree of immunosuppression. The potential for infectious spread into the pleural space and mediastinum can have devastating consequences, making chest wall infections more concerning than other anatomic regional wounds. As cardiothoracic surgery in evermore complex patients continues, especially in the immunosuppressed, chest wall infections are an entity with which the practicing cardiothoracic surgeon must be familiar.

The mainstay of therapy is surgical debridement of devitalized and infected tissue with appropriate antimicrobial administration. Based on extent of tissue resection, deleterious effects on respiratory mechanics may result. The remaining wound bed requires well-vascularized soft tissue coverage if native, healthy tissue is no longer present. Wound management is achieved via negative-pressure wound therapy or chest wall reconstruction, careful to prevent persistence or further spread of infection.

REFERENCES

1. Lim SY, Pyon JK, Mun GH, et al. Reconstructive surgical treatment of tuberculosis abscess in the chest wall. Ann Plast Surg 2010;64(3):302–6.
2. Condos R, Rom WN, Weiden M. Lung-specific immune response in tuberculosis. Int J Tuberc Lung Dis 2000;4(2 Suppl 1):S11–7.
3. Cho S, Lee EB. Surgical resection of chest wall tuberculosis. Thorac Cardiovasc Surg 2009;57(8):480–3.
4. Garg V, Kosmas C, Young PC, et al. Computed tomography-guided percutaneous biopsy for vertebral osteomyelitis: a department's experience. Neurosurg Focus 2014;37(2):E10.
5. Bryan CS, Yarbrough WM. Preventing deep wound infection after coronary artery bypass grafting: a review. Tex Heart Inst J 2013;40(2):125–39.
6. Calhoun JH, Manring MM. Adult osteomyelitis. Infect Dis Clin North Am 2005;19(4):765–86.
7. Ascherman JA, Patel SM, Malhotra SM, et al. Management of sternal wounds with bilateral pectoralis major myocutaneous advancement flaps in 114 consecutively treated patients: refinements in technique and outcomes analysis. Plast Reconstr Surg 2004;114(3):676–83.
8. Abu Arab W, Khadragui I, Echavé V, et al. Surgical management of sternoclavicular joint infection. Eur J Cardiothorac Surg 2011;40(3):630–4.
9. Song HK, Guy TS, Kaiser LR, et al. Current presentation and optimal surgical management of sternoclavicular joint infections. Ann Thorac Surg 2002;73(2):427–31.
10. Chanet V, Soubrier M, Ristori JM, et al. Septic arthritis as a late complication of carcinoma of the breast. Rheumatology (Oxford) 2005;44(9):1157–60.
11. Smith JW, Piercy EA. Infectious arthritis. Clin Infect Dis 1995;20(2):225–30 [quiz: 231].
12. Ross JJ, Shamsuddin H. Sternoclavicular septic arthritis: review of 180 cases. Medicine (Baltimore) 2004;83(3):139–48.

13. Chelli Bouaziz M, Jelassi H, Chaabane S, et al. Imaging of chest wall infections. Skeletal Radiol 2009;38(12):1127–35.

14. Burkhart HM, Deschamps C, Allen MS, et al. Surgical management of sternoclavicular joint infections. J Thorac Cardiovasc Surg 2003;125(4):945–9.

15. Adler BD, Padley SP, Muller NL. Tuberculosis of the chest wall: CT findings. J Comput Assist Tomogr 1993;17(2):271–3.

16. Alton GG, Jones LM, Pietz DE. Laboratory techniques in brucellosis. Monogr Ser World Health Organ 1975;(55):1–163.

17. Gur A, Geyik MF, Dikici B, et al. Complications of brucellosis in different age groups: a study of 283 cases in southeastern Anatolia of Turkey. Yonsei Med J 2003;44(1):33–44.

18. Chernihovski A, Loberant N, Cohen I, et al. Chest wall actinomycosis. Isr Med Assoc J 2007;9(9): 686–7.

19. Mabeza GF, Macfarlane J. Pulmonary actinomycosis. Eur Respir J 2003;21(3):545–51.

20. Bouaddi M, Hassam B. Unusual actinomycosis of the chest wall. Pan Afr Med J 2014;17:61.

21. Kevric I, Cappel MA, Keeling JH. New world and old world leishmania infections: a practical review. Dermatol Clin 2015;33(3):579–93.

22. Dada-Adegbola HO, Oluwatoba OA. Cutaneous myiasis presenting as chronic furunculosis: case report. West Afr J Med 2005;24(4):346–7.

23. Singh A, Singh Z. Incidence of myiasis among humans: a review. Parasitol Res 2015;114(9):3183–99.

24. Steinmetz S, Racloz G, Stern R, et al. Treatment challenges associated with bone echinococcosis. J Antimicrob Chemother 2014;69(3):821–6.

25. Brunetti E, Kern P, Vuitton DA, Writing Panel for the WHO-IWGE. Expert consensus for the diagnosis and treatment of cystic and alveolar echinococcosis in humans. Acta Trop 2010;114(1):1–16.

26. Welvaart WN, Oosterhuis JW, Paul MA. Negative pressure dressing for radiation-associated wound dehiscence after posterolateral thoracotomy. Interact Cardiovasc Thorac Surg 2009;8(5):558–9.

27. Morykwas MJ, Simpson J, Punger K, et al. Vacuum-assisted closure: state of basic research and physiologic foundation. Plast Reconstr Surg 2006;117(7 Suppl):121S–6S.

28. Saxena V, Hwang CW, Huang S, et al. Vacuum-assisted closure: microdeformations of wounds and cell proliferation. Plast Reconstr Surg 2004;114(5): 1086–96 [discussion: 1097–8].

29. Siegel HJ, Long JL, Watson KM, et al. Vacuum-assisted closure for radiation-associated wound complications. J Surg Oncol 2007;96(7):575–82.

30. Damiani G, Pinnarelli L, Sommella L, et al. Vacuum-assisted closure therapy for patients with infected sternal wounds: a meta-analysis of current evidence. J Plast Reconstr Aesthet Surg 2011;64(9): 1119–23.

Thoracoplasty for Tuberculosis in the Twenty-first Century

Denis Krasnov, MD, PhD*, Vladimir Krasnov, MD, PhD,
Dmitry Skvortsov, PhD, Irina Felker, PhD

KEYWORDS

- Pulmonary tuberculosis • Extrapleural thoracoplasty • MDR TB • XDTR TB

KEY POINTS

- A new modification of osteoplastic collapse thoracoplasty performed with a minimally invasive approach has been proposed.
- This operation is a variant of extrapleural thoracoplasty used in the treatment of destructive tuberculosis.
- The benefits of the proposed method, the surgical techniques, and the results of the authors' research are described.
- Compared with the conventional variant of osteoplastic thoracoplasty, the chances of bacteriologic conversion (odds ratio [OR], 1.84; 95% confidence interval [CI], 1.72–1.97) and of the closure of cavities (OR, 2.13; 95% CI, 1.98–2.28) have been proved to be higher when the operation is performed with a minimally invasive approach.

INTRODUCTION

A complicated epidemiologic situation relating to tuberculosis (TB) is currently observed in the Russian Federation. The low efficiency of chemotherapy is confirmed by the number of cases of smear negativity (bacteriologic conversion) in patients with primary pulmonary TB (70%); closure of the decay cavities can be achieved in only 60% of patients with destructive TB. Thus, the number of smear-positive people is growing, jeopardizing the health of the surrounding people: the percentage of smear-positive TB patients reaches 40% of all patients with TB.[1,2]

Because of low compliance with chemotherapy, most such patients should be treated with modern surgical techniques, directed at smear negativity.[3,4] The main operations in the TB surgery are lung resections, designed to remove the main lesion foci.[2–4] However, because of various factors, lung resection may not be performed for all patients; it is contraindicated for many. These factors include the lesion size and its progress, poor lung function, tuberculous lesions of the bronchial tree, and severe concomitant disorders. These patients are smear positive with multidrug-resistant (MDR) TB and extensively drug-resistant (XDR) TB and present a real threat for the community.

Collapse thoracoplasty may be performed on patients with contraindications to lung resection.[4,5] Thoracoplasty has been performed to treat pulmonary TB for more than 100 years and had been successfully used all over the world before invention of the first anti-TB drugs.[5] Using this method has again become a necessity in the countries with a high burden of MRD/XDR TB.

However, the collapse surgical operations developed and described over the preceding decades

Novosibirsk Tuberculosis Research Institute, Federal State Budgetary Institution, Okhotskaya Street 81a, Novosibirsk 630040, Russian Federation
* Corresponding author.
E-mail address: krasnov77@bk.ru

Thorac Surg Clin 27 (2017) 99–111
http://dx.doi.org/10.1016/j.thorsurg.2017.01.003
1547-4127/17/© 2017 Elsevier Inc. All rights reserved.

thoracic.theclinics.com

are accompanied by a large number of complications; an expressed pain syndrome; a significant cosmetic defect; and, as a result, low adherence of patients to this method of treatment.

Therefore, the authors developed and are successfully using a new sparing method of osteoplastic thoracoplasty with a minimally invasive approach that is different from the conventional method in its low degree of invasion, the absence of a cosmetic defect, less intraoperative blood loss, and fewer postoperative complications.

TOPOGRAPHIC-ANATOMIC JUSTIFICATION OF MINIMALLY INVASIVE APPROACH FOR OSTEOPLASTIC THORACOPLASTY

In developing and studying the method of osteoplastic thoracoplasty with a minimally invasive approach, the authors presumed that the approach should be convenient for full-scale surgical intervention and that this impact of the intervention on the patient should be as small as possible. Our study proves the reasonable balance between minimal operative trauma and freedom of access to the posterior chest wall.

In conventional osteoplastic thoracoplasty, the rear segments of the upper 5 ribs and the extrapleural space are approached through a paravertebral incision around the scapular bone, up to 15 to 17 cm long. The trapezoid muscle and the underlying deep muscles of the back are almost completely divided. This approach is convenient because the rear segments of the ribs to be resected are well visualized, and fixation of the ribs to the sixth rib is technically easy after complete extrapleural pneumolysis. Cutting the intercostal muscles of the first and second intercostal spaces allowed surgeons to achieve mobility of the ribs. At the same time, this approach had specific disadvantages. One consisted in cutting the back muscles at length, resulting in serious intraoperative blood loss, the necessity for hemostasis, and the longer operative duration. The operative challenges were later followed by longer confinements for the rehabilitation of patients caused by a severe pain syndrome. A high percentage of purulent processes and hemorrhages in the early postoperative period prolonged the patients' stays in the surgical clinics. The cosmetic defect of the operated patients decreased their adherence to surgical treatment. These factors led us to search for a more sparing approach to this operation and to analyze the possibilities of performing osteoplastic thoracoplasty with a minimally invasive approach.

No studies devoted to objective assessment of approaches used in low-invasive extrapleural thoracoplasty and to their comparison with traditional approaches have been found in the literature. The method of performing osteoplastic thoracoplasty with a minimally invasive approach has not been investigated previously, and the minimal possible sizes of the operative approach have not been justified.

Important criteria for assessing a low-invasive approach are the extent of operative trauma, the view of the operative field, and the universal nature of the approach. In performing osteoplastic thoracoplasty with a minimally invasive approach, the back muscles are traumatized little, which is primarily related to a short incision of 5 cm or less. After dissecting the deep layers of the muscle, visualization of the rear segments of the crossed ribs is not difficult and presents no technical challenges. Installing a rib raspatory makes it easy to view the extrapleural space, which, in its turn, allows the surgeon to mobilize the first rib without any technical confinements. Note that we have refrained from dividing the intercostal muscles in order to reduce intraoperative blood loss and to create conditions for good collapse of the pulmonary tissue. The possibility of fixating the mobilized ribs behind the seventh rib is ensured by making a counteropening in the seventh intercostal space.

This approach to the extrapleural space allows surgeons to exercise direct control over all the anatomic structures of the operative field throughout the intervention, to perform timely homeostasis, and to achieve irreversible circulatory collapse of the pulmonary tissue.

THE SURGICAL TECHNIQUE

A paravertebral approach 4 to 5 cm long is applied to the patient lying in a prone position (**Fig. 1**).

To ensure the convenience of further manipulations, the skin incision is made in the projection of

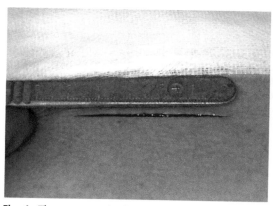

Fig. 1. The paravertebral approach 4 to 5 cm long.

the acanthae of the third and fourth vertebrae. The trapezoid muscle and the deep muscles of the back are cut with an electric coagulator (**Fig. 2**) in the zone of attachment of the upper (I–V) thoracic ribs to the vertebrae.

It is important to remember that it is necessary to leave the upper 3 cm of the trapezoid muscle intact, because this ensures more complete recovery of the function of the upper limb. Then the rear segments of the upper ribs planned for resection are exposed over a length of no more than 3 cm for maximum preservation of the muscles of the first and second intercostal spaces. The rear segment of the third rib is resected intraperiosteally over a length of 3 cm, and extrapleural pneumolysis is begun across its bed toward the first rib (**Fig. 3**).

It is more convenient to start separation with a Kocher probe, later using only blunt tools, a swab, or a finger. To ensure hemostasis, the formed extrapleural space is firmly packed with gauze swabs (**Fig. 4**).

After separation of the lung as far as the spine and from the second rib, the second rib is resected intraperiosteally over a length of 1.5 to 2 cm. Then, after mobilization of the ribs with a Semb raspatory (**Fig. 5**), the underlying ribs IV and V are resected over a length of 8 to 10 cm as far as the posterior axillary line (**Fig. 6**).

The first rib is mobilized as follows. Using an electric coagulator and a rib raspatory, the upper edge of the rib is isolated from the spine to a point located 1 cm alongside the tuberculum musculus scaleni anterior. Near the spine the first intercostal space is cut with an electric coagulator. The raspatory for the first rib is positioned behind the rib near the connection with the spine. The raspatory for the first rib is positioned behind the rib, and the

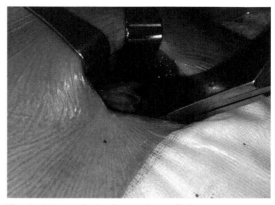

Fig. 3. Intraperiosteal resection of the rear segment of rib III with rib shears Giertz-Stille.

rib is abducted from the subclavicular blood vessels (**Fig. 7**) and is resected near the spine with rib shears (Giertz-Stille or Brunner). The lower stellate ganglion of the sympathetic nerve is attached to the anterior surface of the neck of the first rib and at risk of injury during mobilization and division of the rib. Its impairment may result in development of the Bernard-Horner symptom. Dividing the first rib enlarges the approach to the thoracic cavity and facilitates pneumolysis within the following limits: anterior the limit is the second rib, inferior the seventh intercostal space; medial, it is the mediastinum and fourth or fifth rib; on the left side, the aortal arch serves for orientation.

Lateral pneumolysis is minimized in an effort not to destroy the adhesion between the second and third ribs and the parietal pleura, to later allow additional fixation of the apex of the collapsed lung to the so-called rib module.

The extrapleural space thus formed is firmly filled with gauze swabs. The lung apex is fixated

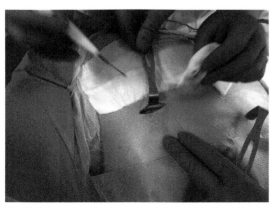

Fig. 2. Dissecting the deep muscles of the back in the projection of the acanthae of ribs III and IV with an electric coagulator.

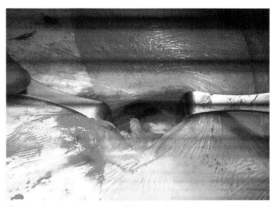

Fig. 4. In the process of formation, the extrapleural space is firmly packed with gauze swabs.

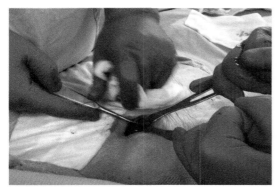

Fig. 5. Mobilization of ribs IV and V with a Semb raspatory.

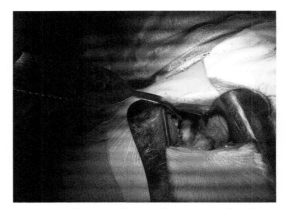

Fig. 7. Mobilization of rib I. The raspatory for rib I is positioned behind the rib near the connection with the spine.

near the vertebra to the sixth, seventh, or eighth ribs. For this purpose, a Billroth grasp is placed on the parietal pleura above the lowered apex of the lung, the pleura above it is sutured with Ethibond, tied under the grasp, raised to the vertebra, and is fixed to the seventh rib by placing this suture through the sixth and seventh intercostal space. Then the ribs are fixed with superdurable nonabsorbable high-density polyethylene by drilling openings at a distance of 1 cm from the edge into the ends of the resected ribs with a surgical awl. Threads are drawn through these openings with a needle (**Fig. 8**).

In order to enhance the collapsing effect of the operation, the rib module of osteoplastic thoracoplasty is formed as follows. At a distance of 4 to 5 cm from the vertebra, in the seventh intercostal space, a forceps of sufficient length is introduced through a puncture in the skin into the extrapleural space (**Fig. 9**), grasping one end of each thread. Then, through the same puncture, the forceps is introduced into the sixth intercostal space, pulling out the second end of each thread. The assistant

pulls the ends of the first, second, and third ribs, one after another under the internal surface of the sixth rib, while the surgeon ties the knots. Thus, the rib module is firmly fixated to the seventh rib, ensuring sufficient collapse of the upper lobe and of partly of the sixth segment of the lung.

Previously, when 5-rib osteoplastic thoracoplasty was used, all the resected ribs were fixated to the sixth rib. The use of the proposed modification allows collapse of the impaired lung segments. A silicon drain is introduced through the skin puncture into the extrapleural space. After hemostasis, the wound is sutured layer by layer (**Fig. 10**). The drain is removed after exudation stops, usually on the third or fourth day after the operation. The mean duration of the operation is, to our knowledge, 50 minutes. The mean intraoperative blood loss was 340 mL.

Thus, this variant of osteoplastic thoracoplasty ensures irreversible selective concentric collapse

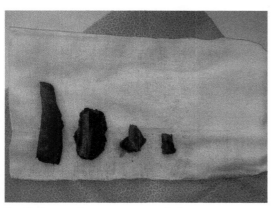

Fig. 6. Resected rear segments of ribs II to IV.

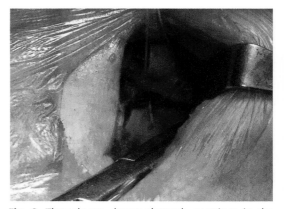

Fig. 8. Threads are drawn through openings in the ends of resected ribs to form a rib module.

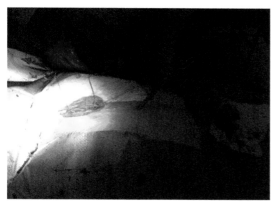

Fig. 9. A forceps is introduced into the extrapleural space through a counteropening in the seventh intercostal space.

of a lung. It is no longer necessary to apply a compressing dressing in the postoperative period, the intervention is not complicated technically, and it does not cause deformity of the chest.

The proposed new method of osteoplastic thoracoplasty with a minimally invasive approach is the operation of choice for patients with destructive pulmonary TB and cavities localized in the upper lobe and the sixth segment of the lung when lung resection is contraindicated or associated with a high risk of severe pleural and pulmonary complications.

INDICATIONS FOR OSTEOPLASTIC THORACOPLASTY

- Single or multiple cavities in the upper lobe with or without superior segmental cavity of 1 or both lungs, with dissemination in the lower divisions or in the opposite lung
- The patient is in a phase of relative stability of TB progression

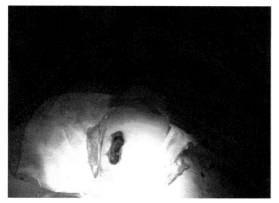

Fig. 10. The postoperative wound before application of sutures layer after layer.

- TB of the tracheobronchial tree
- Limited functional reserve excludes the possibility of resection

CONTRAINDICATIONS FOR OSTEOPLASTIC THORACOPLASTY

- Total fibrocavernous TB or caseous pneumonia as a result of TB process progression
- Cachexia
- Respiratory insufficiency III (the Medical Research Council [MRC] scale) or cardiovascular decompensation
- Amyloidosis of internal organs with functional impairment
- Combination of the TB process with bronchiectasis or abscess in the lower lobe of the same lung
- Concomitant diseases with poor prognosis

CLINICAL OUTCOMES

A prospective cohort trial was held in the thoracic clinic of the Novosibirsk Tuberculosis Institute. The trial started in January 2007. It ended in December 2013.

The results assessed in the clinical trial included the clinical and laboratory parameters comparing patients undergoing minimally invasive osteoplastic thoracoplasty with conventional osteoplastic thoracoplasty. The following criteria were applied: smear negativity and closure of the decay cavities in the lungs. The volume of intraoperative blood loss was assessed, as well as the postoperative complications that occurred.

Direct results of the surgical treatment were evaluated with the patients under study 12 and 18 months after the osteoplastic thoracoplasty, based on the clinical data, radiograph images, and laboratory tests. The following categories of the results were chosen: considerable improvement, improvement, deterioration of the condition, and death.

Considerable improvement was defined as elimination of abscess cavities and bacteriologic conversion of patients. The category of improvement included patients whose general condition normalized, in whom sepsis resolved, whose smear became negative or the amount of purulent sputum decreased, in whom dissemination and perifocal inflammatory foci fully or partly resolved, and the size of the cavities decreased. The category of deterioration was defined as postoperative clinical progression of the infection.

The results 2 to 4 years after osteoplastic thoracoplasty were analyzed. The intermediate-term results of surgical treatment were evaluated from the clinical cure criteria, of formation of a chronic process, progress of TB, and death.

The criteria for including patients were:

- Age from 18 to 70 years.
- Clinically and radiologically confirmed signs of destructive pulmonary TB, with cavities localized in the upper lobe or in the upper lobe and the sixth segment of the lower lobe of 1 or both lungs. After previous upper lobectomy, a patient could be involved in the study if there were lower lobe cavities, at the discretion of the researcher.
- Dyspnea grade 1 to 4 (the MRC Dyspnea Scale), grade 0 to 2 respiratory insufficiency (the degree of severity scale).
- The patient read, understood, and signed the informed consent form.

Criteria for excluding a patient from the trial:

- Location of cavities in the lower lobe of the lung, except for the cases indicated in item 2 of the inclusion criteria.
- Bilateral total destructive TB (both lungs are destroyed).
- Dyspnea grade 5 (the MRC Dyspnea Scale), respiratory insufficiency grade 3 (classification by the degree of severity), and/or pulmonary and cardiac insufficiency with decompensation signs.
- Pregnancy or lactation.
- Charlson Comorbidity Index greater than 6.
- Empyema of the pleura.
- Body mass index less than 16 and/or cachexia.
- Combination of the TB process with bronchiectasia or an abscess in the lower lobe of the same lung.

In accordance with these criteria, 414 patients with destructive pulmonary TB were involved in the trial (**Table 1**). The main group consisted of 191 patients; of these, 105 were diagnosed with pulmonary TB more than 2 years before enrollment in the trial and 86 less than 2 years. The control group consisted of 223 patients.

By the time of admission to the surgical department, all the patients had destructive TB, with bilateral cavities in 43 (22.5% ± 3.0%) patients of the study group and 61 patients (27.4% ± 3.0%) of the control group ($P = .26$, χ^2). Radiological signs of continuous progression of pericavitary infiltrates with extensive dissemination of bacteria in the lung segments in most patients were present in 167 (87.4% ± 2.4%) patients in the study group and 179 (80.3% ± 2.7%) patients in the control group. The TB process in the other patients was

Table 1
Distribution of patients by groups in accordance with the treatment provided

Group of Patients	Treatment
The main group (group 1) (n = 191)	Osteoplastic thoracoplasty performed with a minimally invasive approach; a personalized regimen of anti-TB therapy based on the drug resistance test results
The control group (group 2) (n = 223)	Conventional osteoplastic thoracoplasty; a personalized regimen of anti-TB therapy based on the drug resistance test results

evaluated as unstable with frequent exacerbations in 24 study (12.6% ± 2.4%) and 44 control (19.7% ± 2.7%) patients ($P = .05$, χ^2).

Cavities were most often found in the upper lobe or in the upper lobe and the superior segment of the lower lobes. Cavities in the lower lobe of those patients in whom upper lobectomies were previously performed were found in 13 study (6.8% ± 1.8%) and 19 control (8.5% ± 1.9%) patients ($P = .52$, χ^2). Multiple cavernous lesions of the lung tissue (2 or more cavities) were found in 118 (61.8% ± 3.5%) patients of the study group and 138 (61.9% ± 3.3%) patients of the control group ($P = .98$, χ^2). Bilateral subtotal dissemination of bacteria in the lungs was found in 178 (93.2% ± 1.8%) and 213 (95.5% ± 1.4%) cases ($P = .30$, χ^2), new infiltrates were found in the opposite lung in 39 study (20.4% ± 2.9%) and 42 control (18.8% ± 2.6%) patients ($P = .69$, χ^2).

Despite the specific intense chemotherapy, bacterial sputum excretion persisted before the operation in 179 study (93.7% ± 1.8%) and 207 control (92.8% ± 1.7%) patients ($P = .72$, χ^2) and was massive in 120 study (67.1% ± 3.5%) and 145 control (70.1% ± 3.2%) smear-positive patients ($P = .53$, χ^2). Among the patients with drug resistance of the pathogen, MDR was found in most: in the study group in 136 (88.9% ± 2.5%) and in the control group in 161 (86.1% ± 2.5%) patients ($P = .44$, χ^2). MDR was recorded in 71.2% ± 3.2% study cases and in 72.2% ± 3.0% controls ($P = .82$, χ^2). In more than half of the patients with drug resistance of the pathogen, extensively drug-resistant TB was observed in 99 study (64.7% ± 3.9%) and 106 control (56.7% ± 3.6%) patients ($P = .13$, χ^2).

Because of the abundance of the process in the lungs and the commonly occurring concomitant chronic obstructive pulmonary disease (COPD), manifestations of respiratory insufficiency were observed in a significant number of the patients in both groups. The main parameters of respiratory function complied with the normal values only in 44 (23.1% ± 3.1%) and 45 (20.2% ± 2.7%) patients ($P = .48$, χ^2). Concomitant COPD was found in 32 (16.8% ± 2.7%) cases in the first group and in 51 (22.9% ± 2.8%) cases in the control group ($P = .12$, χ^2).

Impairment of the tracheobronchial tree is an important factor compromising the severity of the condition of the observed patients. Purulent endobronchitis was diagnosed in 142 study (74.3% ± 3.2%) cases and 159 controls (71.3% ± 3.0%), rendering the surgical method difficult and essentially prolonging the duration of the preoperative preparation period ($P = .49$, χ^2). Specific impairment of the tracheobronchial tree was found in 112 study cases (58.6% ± 3.6%) and 110 controls (49.3% ± 3.4%) ($P = .06$, χ^2), indicating a contraindication to resection.

Thus, the most difficult patients with destructive pulmonary TB were included in the study, and those who had an unstable and wavelike process with frequent exacerbations causing continuous progress of the disease were found in both groups. No notable preoperative differences were found among patients from both groups. Persistent sepsis, intense bacterial excretion, specific impairment of the tracheobronchial tree, and signs of respiratory insufficiency determined inadequacy of the specific chemotherapy administered to the patients and accounted for contraindications to resection surgery. Under the existing conditions, the osteoplastic collapse thoracoplasty proved to be the operation of choice selected among the available surgical assistance methods.

A total of 196 osteoplastic collapse thoracoplasty operations were performed on the patients of the main group, whereas 238 such operations were performed on the patients of the control group; bilateral surgical operations were performed on 5 (2.6% ± 1.2%) patients of the first group and on 15 (6.7% ± 1.7%) patients of the second group ($P = .05$, χ^2). In both groups, the 5-rib variant of the operation prevailed: in 159 (81.1% ± 2.8%) and 205 (86.1% ± 2.2%) cases ($P = .16$, χ^2).

COMPLICATIONS AND CONCERNS

Osteoplastic thoracoplasty with a minimally invasive approach reduced intraoperative blood loss to 400 mL in 187 (95.4% ± 1.5%) patients in the study group. In patients operated with the conventional approach, intraoperative blood loss of less than 400 mL occurred in 105 (44.1% ± 3.2%) cases ($P = .0001$, χ^2) (relative risk [RR], 10.10; 95% CI, 9.20–11.01). Significant intraoperative blood loss (>500 mL) occurred in 1 (0.5% ± 0.5%) case of the main group and in 69 (29.0% ± 2.9%) patients of the control group ($P = .0001$, χ^2). Mean intraoperative blood loss during osteoplastic thoracoplasty was 278 ± 20 mL in the study group and 438 ± 22 mL among controls ($P<.05$).

Traumatic pneumothorax was the only intraoperative complication occurring in 10 study (5.1% ± 1.6%) and 28 control (11.8% ± 2.1%) cases ($P = .05$, χ^2). Traumatic pneumothorax was eliminated by drainage, ensuring a favorable outcome of the operation, so the operative plan was not changed.

The postoperative course was complicated in 28 study (14.7% ± 2.6%) patients of the first group and in 69 control (30.9% ± 3.1%) patients ($P = .0001$, χ^2). The risk of complications in the early postoperative period in doing osteoplastic thoracoplasty using a conventional approach was higher (RR, 1.46; 95% CI, 1.38–1.54). Severe complications, such as hemorrhage into the extrapleural space, an extensive postoperative wound infection, progression of TB followed by respiratory insufficiency, and hypostatic pneumonia, occurred in 14 study patients (7.3% ± 1.9%) and 49 controls (22.0% ± 2.9%) of the groups under study ($P = .0001$, χ^2).

An extensive wound infection originating from the extrapleural zone took place in 3 study (1.6% ± 0.9%) and 5 control (2.2% ± 1.0%) patients ($P = .45$, Fisher exact test). These wounds were managed with irrigation and removal of the fragments of resected ribs. The outcome of these complications was positive.

In 1 study (0.5% ± 0.5%) and 10 control (4.5% ± 1.4%) cases ($P = .01$, Fisher exact test), postoperative drainage revealed hemorrhage in the extrapleural space: operative exploration by thoracotomy was performed in all patients. In all cases, diffuse bleeding was found from the cavity walls, whereas there was no hemorrhage from the large vessels. In most patients, hemorrhage was stopped by using modern hemostatic approaches and means; in 2 control cases continuing hemorrhage required local application of swabs in the remaining extrapleural space and irrigation with 5% solution of the ε-amino caproic acid. The swabs were removed on the second or third day. The hemorrhage did not recur.

In 8 study (4.2% ± 1.5%) and 12 control (5.4% ± 1.5%) cases, postoperative pneumonia was found in the operated lung (P = .37, Fisher exact test). The use of inhalation therapy, wide-spectrum antibiotics, and postural drainage enabled successful treatment of the complications in all cases.

Progressive pulmonary TB accompanied by respiratory insufficiency occurred after osteoplastic thoracoplasty in 6 cases of the study group (3.1% ± 1.3%) and 22 control cases (9.9% ± 2.0%) (P = .005, Fisher exact test). Correction of the anti-TB therapy ensured stabilization of the process in 2 cases in the main group and in 11 cases in the control group.

Thus, statistically relevant differences were found between the groups for the rate of postoperative hemorrhage (P = .01, Fisher exact test) and postprocedure progression of disease (P = .005, Fisher exact test). Postoperative complications were avoided in 85.7% ± 6.6% of study cases and in 84.0% ± 4.4% of controls (P = .84, χ^2).

Further, a valvular bronchial blocker was placed after thoracoplasty in most patients of both groups[6]: 163 (85.3% ± 2.6%) and 191 (85.7% ± 2.4%) (P = .93, χ^2); there were few complications after this procedure, and they were removed easily.

OUTCOME OF THE STUDY

The early outcome was evaluated 12 and 18 months after the operation, and the intermediate-term outcome after 2 to 4 years.

The use of minimally invasive osteoplastic thoracoplasty was associated with bacteriologic conversion in 144 (80.4% ± 2.9%) cases 12 months after the surgery. Among patients with conventional osteoplastic thoracoplasty, bacteriologic conversion was recorded for 124 (69.3% ± 3.5%) cases (P = .01, χ^2; OR, 1.84; 95% CI, 1.72–1.97).

During the first year after thoracoplasty, closure of the decay cavities was observed in 159 (83.2% ± 2.7%) study cases with minimally invasive osteoplastic thoracoplasty; frequently at a higher rate than in the conventional group, with 156 cases (70.0% ± 3.0%; P = .002, χ^2; OR, 2.13; 95% CI, 1.98–2.28).

Further broad-spectrum anti-TB treatment was provided in 6 study (3.1% ± 1.3%) and 9 control (4.0% ± 1.3%) cases (P = .45, Fisher exact test), showing the efficiency of osteoplastic thoracoplasty. At 18 months after surgery, 173 (90.6% ± 2.1%) study patients were reported to have considerable improvement of their condition, whereas 14 (7.3% ± 1.9%) study cases had an improved condition. In the control group, these figures are statistically notably lower: considerable improvement was observed in 176 (78.9% ± 2.8%) patients (P = .001, χ^2) and improvement was recorded in 35 (15.8% ± 2.4%) patients (P = .009, χ^2) (**Table 2**).

Clinical cure of TB treated with minimally invasive osteoplastic thoracoplasty was observed in the intermediate term in 169 (88.5% ± 2.3%) study cases and 179 (79.7% ± 2.7%) controls (P = .016, χ^2) (**Table 3**).

Thus, comprehensive treatment including surgical collapse therapy with minimally invasive osteoplastic thoracoplasty increased the chances of achieving clinical cure (OR, 1.09; 95% CI, 1.05–1.12), compared with the conventional surgery.

The authors emphasize that these intermediate-term results occurred in a difficult category of patients having severe clinical manifestations of the disease and unstable course of the process, who had problems with adherence to chemotherapy and who presented a high epidemiologic hazard for the community.

A CLINICAL CASE STUDY

As an example of the surgical treatment of a case with bilateral progressing destructive TB using bilateral stepwise 5-rib minimally invasive

---

Table 2
Results of treatment 18 months after the surgery

| Results | Group of Patients | | | | | |
| | 1 Group | | 2 Group | | | |
	n	%	n	%	P
Considerable improvement	173	90.6 ± 2.1	176	78.9 ± 2.8	.001[a]
Improvement	14	7.3 ± 1.9	35	15.8 ± 2.4	.009[a]
Deterioration	4	2.1 ± 1.0	11	4.9 ± 1.5	.2[b]
Death	0	0.0 ± 0.0	1	0.4 ± 0.5	—
Total cases	191	100	223	100	—

[a] Pearson χ^2.
[b] Fisher exact test.

Table 3
Results of treatment of 2 to 4 years after osteoplastic thoracoplasty

| | Group of Patients | | | | |
| | 1 Group | | 2 Group | | |
Results	n	%	n	%	P
Clinical cure	169	88.5 ± 2.3	177	79.7 ± 2.7	.016[a]
Formation of a chronic process	15	7.9 ± 2.0	30	13.5 ± 2.3	.066[a]
Progress of TB	6	3.1 ± 1.3	13	5.9 ± 1.6	.14[b]
Death	1	0.5 ± 0.5	2	0.9 ± 0.6	.56[b]
Total cases	191	100	222	100	—

[a] Pearson χ^2.
[b] Fisher exact test.

osteoplastic thoracoplasties on both sides, with subsequent bilateral valvular blocking of the upper lobe bronchi and the left B6 bronchus, this article presents the following case (**Figs. 11 and 12**).

Patient K, 44 years of age, was first diagnosed and put on the TB record with disseminated pulmonary TB complicated by left pleuritis in 1996. Treatment was conducted according to 1 regimen (isoniazid [H], rifampicin [R], ethambutol [E], streptomycin [S]), with multiple pleural punctures in a hospital and lasted 6 months, when the patient was switched to the continuation regimen. In 2000, the patient was taken off the TB record. In 2010, the patient was diagnosed in Italy with left-side spontaneous pneumothorax and drainage of the left pleural cavity was performed. After expansion of the lung, the radiological examination revealed a relapse of pulmonary TB and chemotherapy was administered. In 2011, the patient's smear was found to be positive, and linezolid was added to the treatment plan. Despite treatment, the disease progressed, and in 2013 the patient returned to Russia to continue treatment. In March 2013, multiple drug resistance was found to H, R, E, S, and kanamycin (K). Fourth-regimen treatment started; the patient's smear negativity occurred 4 months after, and, beginning in July 2013,

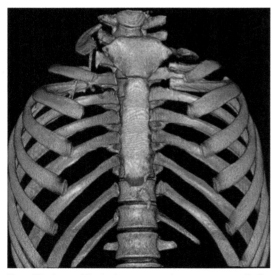

Fig. 11. A multispiral computed tomogram of the lungs of patient K after bilateral osteoplastic thoracoplasties. Three-dimensional (3D) modeling of the chest, front shot.

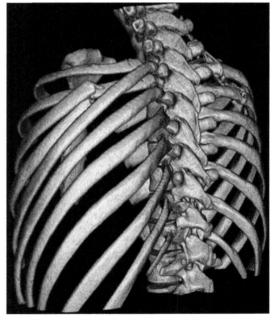

Fig. 12. A multispiral computed tomogram of the lungs of patient K after bilateral osteoplastic thoracoplasties. 3D modeling of the chest, shot from behind.

the patient was treated for TB on a walk-in basis. The examination conducted in October 2013 revealed exacerbation of TB and a positive smear, with destructive malformations preserved. After a consultation, the patient was admitted to the surgical clinic of the Novosibirsk Tuberculosis Institute on November 2, 2013, to be further examined and possibly to be operated. During the admittance procedure, the patient complained of cough with scanty sputum and dyspnea at exercise. His breathing was vesicular, harsh, and weakened in the upper parts of the lungs. His body temperature was normal. His blood pressure was 120/70 mm Hg and the respiratory rate was 20 breaths per minute.

The radiograph (**Fig. 13**) showed an enlarged right lung. There were emphysematous-bullous changes and fibrosis, more intense in the upper lobe and in S6. The upper lobe was reduced in volume with a deformed cavity 59 ч 25 mm in the axial projection, fused over a considerable length with the thickened pleura. There were adjacent different foci of the infection and calcifications. In the middle and lower lobes, there were multiple foci of infection without signs of perifocal infiltrates, calcifications, and small accumulations of conglomerates in S6. In the left lung, the upper lobe and S6 had a significantly reduced volume with reduced aeration, primarily caused by cirrhotic changes, fused with

thickened and dense apical and costal pleura. In the upper lobe there were clear contours of 2 deformed cavities at a small distance from each other: their sizes were 36 mm and 35 mm. There may have been small cavities in the end parts of the bronchi. In S6, paracostally on the dorsal surface, there was a deformed cavity, with its shape approaching that of a fissure in the axial projection and its size being 58 ч 7 mm. In the basal parts of the lower lobe, with fibrous and bullous-emphysematous lesions, there were many foci of various sizes and calcifications. There was a 10-mm cavity on the border of S9 and S10. The long roots were deformed and lifted, the left root had an unclear structure because of involvement of its structures at the level of the left upper lobe bronchus, B6, into the apneumatosis zone. The bronchi were deformed on both sides; the deformity was greater in the upper lobes and on the left S6. The bronchial walls were dense and thickened. There was no fluid in the pleural cavities. The sinus was obliterated on the left. The cupulas of the diaphragm had commissural fibers on both sides. The mediastinum was shifted to the left side.

Bronchoscopy showed bilateral diffuse atrophic endobronchitis of the first degree of inflammation. There was restricted purulent endobronchitis of the left upper lobe bronchus of the second degree of inflammation, B1 to B2, B3. There were endoscopic signs of TB of the left upper lobe bronchus,

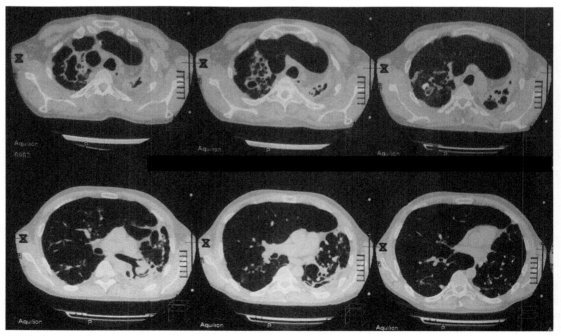

Fig. 13. A multispiral computed tomogram of the lungs of patient K before surgical treatment. The slice thickness is 5 mm.

B1 to B2, B3, with infiltrates with stenosis of the second degree.

On the spirographic test, the lung capacity was essentially reduced (close to the boundary with the norm). There was significant impairment of bronchial patency. The ventilating ability of the lungs was sharply decreased.

The electrocardiogram (ECG), showed sinus tachycardia, and heart rate was 112 beats per minute; after breathing in, there was an episode of sinus arrhythmia with the heart rate 63 to 92 beats per minute. There was a sequence on the right crus of the His band. There were signs of hypertrophy of the left atrium and of the right ventricle. There were moderate diffuse changes in the myocardium. There was electric alternation of QRS in the chest leads.

Doppler-ECG with color flow Doppler imaging showed impairment of the diastolic function of the left and right ventricles as slow relaxation. The heart valves were normal. There was first-degree regurgitation on the valve of the pulmonary artery and first-degree regurgitation on the tricuspid valve. Pulmonary hypertension could not be excluded.

Complete blood count results were: erythrocytes 4.56×10^{12}/L; hemoglobin level, 134 g/L; erythrocyte sedimentation rate, 35 mm/h; leukocytes 8.34×10^9/L; eosinophil level, 3%; stabs (band neutrophils or stab cells), 5%; segmented neutrophil level, 57%; lymphocyte level, 30%; monocyte level, 5%.

Microscopy of the sputum smear revealed from 1 to 10 visible acid-resistant mycobacteria. The diagnosis was progressing fibrous-cavernous pulmonary TB in the phase of infiltrates and dissemination; TB of the upper lobe bronchus, B1 to 2, B3; infiltrates; *Mycobacterium tuberculosis* plus MDR (H, R, E, S, K). A complication was respiratory insufficiency, degree 2. A concomitant diagnosis was COPD, at the stage of unstable remission.

Considering the presence of a large cavity in the upper lobe of the right lung, a cavity in the upper lobe, and a large cavity in S6 in the left lung, and the active nature of the process with specific lesion of the tracheobronchial tree and persistent massive excretion of MDR *M tuberculosis*, the physicians and medical researchers of the institute decided to administer stepwise surgical treatment to the patient: 5-rib osteoplastic thoracoplasty of the left lung, with subsequent installation of an endobronchial valve in the left upper lobe bronchus and the left B6, and, a month later, 5-rib osteoplastic thoracoplasty of the right lung, with subsequent installation of an endobronchial valve in the right upper lobe bronchus.

The first operation was conducted applying a minimally invasive approach on November 7, 2013 (**Fig. 14**). The operation lasted 45 minutes,

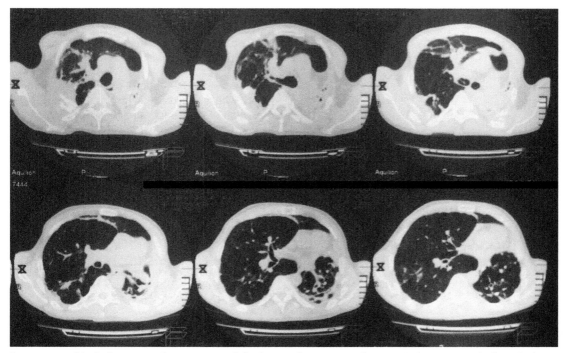

Fig. 14. A multispiral computed tomogram of the lungs of patient K after surgical treatment before discharge from the hospital. The scan confirms closure of the cavities in both lungs.

and the intraoperative blood loss was 250 mL. The postoperative period was easy. The drain was removed on the fifth day after the operation. On November 13, 2013, a valvular bronchial blocker was installed in the left upper lobe bronchus and in the left B6 under general anesthesia.

The patient continued anti-TB treatment in the surgical department of the institute for 4 weeks. He was examined before the next phase of the surgical treatment: no deviations in the clinical tests were found. His external respiration function was tested: bronchial patency deteriorated, the forced expiratory volume in 1 second decreased by 27% from the actual value, and the lung capacity decreased by 23% from the actual value.

Five-rib osteoplastic thoracoplasty of the right lung was performed with a minimally invasive approach on December 5, 2013 (**Figs. 14 and 15**). The operation lasted 45 minutes, and the intraoperative blood loss was 200 mL. The postoperative period was easy. The drain was removed on the fourth day after the operation. On December 12, 2013, a valvular bronchial blocker was installed in the right upper lobe bronchus under general anesthesia.

Further, the patient was treated in the therapeutic department of the local TB dispensary. The period of temporary occlusion since installation of the first endobronchial valve was 12 months. The radiological control examination did not show any destructive changes in the collapsed parts of both lungs. The patient's smear became negative 5 months after the operation.

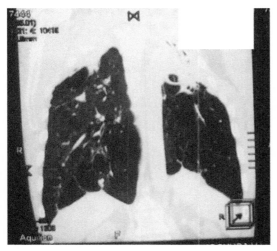

Fig. 15. A multispiral computed tomogram of the lungs of patient K after surgical treatment before discharge from the hospital. The scan confirms closure of the cavities in both lungs.

In summary, bilateral 5-rib osteoplastic thoracoplasties were performed with a minimally invasive approach in combination with installation of a valvular bronchial blocker in the upper lobe bronchi on both sides and in B6 on the left side for a patient with progressing destructive TB of both lungs with massive excretion of MDR *M tuberculosis* with second-degree respiratory insufficiency and COPD, the prolonged conservative treatment of whom had been ineffective. A complete clinical effect was achieved: smear negativity and elimination of destructive changes.

SUMMARY

The novel sparing technique of performing osteoplastic thoracoplasty developed by the authors allows all the stages of the operation to be performed with a minimally invasive approach of 5 cm or less under direct visual control of all the surrounding anatomic structures and achieving the required selective concentric collapse of the lung tissue in patients with destructive pulmonary TB.

The proposed tactic of comprehensive surgical treatment reduces the rates of intraoperative blood loss greater than 400 mL (RR, 10.10; 95% CI, 9.20–11.01) and of postoperative complications (RR, 1.46; 95% CI, 1.38–1.54).

The chances of achieving smear negativity (OR, 1.84; 95% CI, 1.72–1.97) of closure of the decay cavities (OR, 2.13; 95% CI, 1.98–2.28) in performing osteoplastic thoracoplasty with a minimally invasive approach are reliably higher.

The developed method of osteoplastic thoracoplasty with a minimally invasive approach is the operation of choice for surgical collapse intervention in cases of destructive pulmonary TB, because the chance of achieving clinical cure in patients 2 to 4 years after the surgery are higher (OR, 1.09; 95% CI, 1.05–1.12).

REFERENCES

1. The Ministry of Health of the Russian Federation. Tuberculosis in the Russian Federation, 2011. Analytical review of statistical parameters used in the Russian Federation and abroad. Moscow (Russia): 2013. p. 280. Available at: http://mednet.ru/images/stories/files/CMT/tbreview2011.pdf. Accessed June 13, 2016.
2. Yablonsky PK, Sokolovich EG, Avetisyan AO, et al. The role of thoracic surgery in the treatment of pulmonary tuberculosis (literature review and the authors' observations). Med Alliance J 2014;3:4–10 [in Russian].

3. Rare operations in thoracic surgery. Edited by corresponding member of the Russian Academy of Medical Sciences Prof. Yu. N. Levashev. St Petersburg (Russia): Aurora-Design; 2010. p. 188.

4. World Health Organization. The role of surgery in the treatment of pulmonary TB and multidrug- and extensively drug-resistant TB. World Health Organization, 2014. p. 17. Available at: http://www.euro.who.int/__data/assets/pdf_file/0005/259691/The-role-of-surgery-in-the-treatment-of-pulmonary-TB-and-multidrug-and-extensively-drug-resistant-TB.pdf?ua=1. Accessed June 15, 2016.

5. Barker WL. Thoracoplasty. Chest Surg Clin North America 1994;4(3):593–615.

6. Levin AV, Tseimakh EA, Zimonin PE. The application of a valvular bronchial blocker in combination with thoracoplasties in complex treatment of patients with pulmonary tuberculosis with multiple drug resistance. Bull East Siberian Res Cent Siberian branch Russ Acad Med Sci 2011;2(78):64–6.http://www.medlung.ru.

Chest Wall Trauma

Sarah Majercik, MD, MBA[a],*, Fredric M. Pieracci, MD, MPH[b]

KEYWORDS

- Chest trauma • Rib fractures • Flail chest • Surgical stabilization of rib fractures

KEY POINTS

- Chest wall trauma causes significant morbidity and mortality in injured patients.
- Adequate analgesia for patients with severe rib fractures/flail chest is critical. Locoregional modalities are more effective than oral or parenteral opioids.
- Mechanical ventilation should be used for pulmonary dysfunction. Noninvasive ventilation strategies are effective.
- Surgical stabilization of severe rib fractures is beneficial in the short and long term, and should be considered in select patients.

INTRODUCTION

Chest wall trauma is common. Approximately half a million patients presented to emergency departments in the United States in 2013 with an injury to their bony thorax, and about 200,000 of those were hospitalized.[1] Reported morbidity and mortality rates after chest wall injury vary widely, but clearly increase with age and number of rib fractures.[2–5] Flail chest, generally defined as three or more ribs fractured in two or more places, carries an even higher risk of mortality,[6] and many patients who sustain flail chest suffer from long-term pain, disability, and inability to maintain employment.[7–10] Patients with flail chest often have significant pulmonary contusion, which further contributes to short- and long-term morbidity and mortality.[11,12] Although many patients who suffer chest wall trauma also have injury to soft tissue and intrathoracic structures, this article focuses on bony injuries of the ribs and sternum.

HISTORICAL PERSPECTIVE

Diagnosis and management of chest wall injury has been described as far back as 3000 BC.[13] The first modern descriptions of "stove in chest" and flail chest were published in 1945[14] and 1955,[15] respectively. Throughout the 1960s and 1970s, patients with severe chest wall trauma were managed with "internal pneumatic stabilization,"[16,17] or long-term positive pressure mechanical ventilation. In 1976, Trinkel and colleagues[18] and Shackford and colleagues[19] challenged this notion, and since that time, mechanical ventilation has been used as appropriate for pulmonary dysfunction and to correct abnormalities of gas exchange, but not as a "stabilizing" agent per se.

Over the past century, various surgical methods for repairing rib fractures have been described.[20] Despite these descriptions, treatment of severe chest wall injury has remained largely nonsurgical.[6] In the past two decades, there has been a sharp

Disclosure Statement: Dr S. Majercik has nothing to disclose. Dr F.M. Pieracci has received financial research support from DePuy Synthes (45007100), makers of the MatrixRIB fixation system.
[a] Division of Trauma and Surgical Critical Care, Intermountain Medical Center, 5121 South Cottonwood Street, Murray, UT 84107, USA; [b] Department of Surgery, Denver Health Medical Center, University of Colorado School of Medicine, 777 Bannock Street, MC0206, Denver, CO 80204, USA
* Corresponding author.
E-mail address: Sarah.majercik@imail.org

thoracic.theclinics.com

increase in interest in the surgical stabilization of rib fractures (SSRF), with several authors showing improved outcomes compared with conventional management in the most severely injured patients.[21–24] Medical device manufacturers have developed and marketed various rib-specific fixation systems, and use of surgical techniques has grown. Surgical and nonsurgical management strategies are discussed in this article.

MECHANISMS OF INJURY

In the civilian world, most injuries to the chest wall result from blunt injury. The most common mechanism of injury is motor vehicle crash, followed by pedestrians struck by vehicles, falls, and crush injuries.[25,26]

ANATOMIC CONSIDERATIONS

The ribs, sternum, clavicles, scapulae, and vertebrae are the major bony structures that comprise the chest wall. Because of the amount of energy required to fracture these bones, one must always have a heightened index of suspicion that there is underlying thoracic or abdominal visceral injury when a bony chest wall fracture is discovered.[24,27,28] An exception to this is in the elderly, where the bones are less strong, and thus, often fracture after low-energy incidents.[29] In children, rib fractures are less common because of increased compliance of the thoracic cage. Thus, if a child does sustain a fractured rib, one must have a high suspicion of severe intrathoracic or abdominal injuries.[30]

INITIAL MANAGEMENT

Identification of major chest wall and intrathoracic injuries figure prominently in the initial management, or "primary survey"[31] of the multiply injured trauma patient. After attending to the airway, breathing, and circulation, a history should be taken if possible, and physical examination focused on diagnosis of life-threating conditions rapidly performed. With specific regard to the chest wall, the examiner should observe chest rise, looking for areas of obvious asymmetry that may suggest a flail segment. The chest wall can also be palpated, with the examiner feeling for symmetry, crepitance, or perhaps mobile segments of the chest wall. Although difficult in a noisy emergency department setting, auscultation should also be performed.

In the hemodynamically stable patient with severe chest wall injury with suspected pulmonary contusion, one should be judicious with crystalloid fluid resuscitation. Although the evidence is not strong that volume of crystalloid correlates with eventual outcomes,[32] it is prudent to avoid unnecessary intravenous fluid administration.

RADIOGRAPHIC DIAGNOSIS

An anteroposterior plain chest radiograph (CXR) is still an important initial study to obtain in a major trauma patient in whom one suspects major thoracic injury, simply because it can rapidly diagnose immediately life-threatening intrathoracic pathology, such as tension pneumothorax or massive hemothorax. The endotracheal tube position can be checked, and the clinician can evaluate the pleural spaces, the mediastinum, and bones for obvious injuries. It is well-documented, however, that CXR has low sensitivity for diagnosing rib fractures and some serious intrathoracic pathology, such as pulmonary contusion.[33] Computed tomography (CT) of the chest is commonly (perhaps too commonly) used in trauma patients as a more sensitive test to definitively diagnose chest wall and/or intrathoracic injury. The CT can provide much more precise injury information, but care should be taken not to use it indiscriminately. There are published decision rules/algorithms[34,35] to help clinicians decide when chest CT is warranted. Most use a combination of patient and injury criteria that are predictors for significant thoracic injury. In cases where multiple rib fractures are suspected or diagnosed by CXR, chest CT has become standard practice to characterize all of the chest wall/intrathoracic injuries, and to evaluate whether surgical repair of the ribs is warranted.[21,24]

MANAGEMENT OF CHEST WALL INJURIES
Rib Fractures/Flail Chest

The management of patients with multiple, displaced rib fractures or flail chest consists of three basic tenets: (1) pain management, (2) management of pulmonary dysfunction, and (3) surgical fixation. Previous authors have shown that multidisciplinary protocols or clinical pathways for managing patients with multiple rib fractures yields better clinical results,[36,37] including decreased mortality, decreased pneumonia, shorter hospital and intensive care unit length of stay,[38] and less return visits to the emergency department.[39] This was found to be particularly true for patients who are older than 65.[36] Development and implementation of a clinical pathway should be considered at institutions that treat patients with severe chest wall trauma with any regularity.

Pain Management

Pain control in the immediate postinjury period is of the utmost importance in patients with severe chest wall injury. Ideally, the patient should be kept comfortable enough that he or she can deep breathe, cough, and participate in pulmonary toilet exercises, and ambulate as much as possible. Although parenteral or oral opioids are an obvious and simple choice from the clinician's point of view, one should keep in mind that locoregional modalities may be more effective,[40,41] and avoid putting the patient at risk for long-term narcotic dependence. The most common locoregional modalities currently in use are discussed next.

Lidocaine patches

In one randomized study[42] of patients with rib fractures, use of a lidocaine patch did not affect total in-hospital intravenous opioid usage. Another retrospective study[43] found similar results with regard to opioids, but did report that patients who received the patch had decreased pain scores. Lidocaine patches have a benign risk profile, and can continue to be used after hospital discharge.

Thoracic epidural catheters

Epidural is the most well-studied mode of locoregional pain control. In patients with multiple rib fractures, epidural has been shown to result in lower mortality,[44,45] lower pain scores,[46] improved pulmonary function,[45,47] and decreased pneumonia rates[48] compared with other modalities. One group found that patients with an epidural experienced higher rates of venous thromboembolism than did those without an epidural.[49] Epidural placement is somewhat complex, because it requires coordination with the anesthesia pain service, normal conventional coagulation tests, and no spine fracture. Furthermore, epidural does carry with it the risks of cardiac arrest, neurologic injury, headache, urinary retention, infection, and hematoma.[50]

Intercostal nerve blocks with or without a continuous infusion catheter

Intercostal nerve blocks as a "single shot"[51] or with a continuous infusion catheter have been shown to be as effective as epidural anesthesia,[52] and may decrease hospital stay and ventilator days and improve pain scores.[53] Intercostal blocks have the advantage of being able to be used in patients with coagulopathy and those with spine fractures. Furthermore, they have been shown to be easily placed in the emergency department,[45] thus avoiding involving the anesthesia pain service.

Management of Pulmonary Dysfunction

After severe chest wall injury, patients can experience acute, significant pulmonary dysfunction. This may be caused by the loss of respiratory mechanical function from the flail chest or an underlying pulmonary contusion. Inadequate pain management hinders deep breathing and coughing/secretion clearance. Later on in the hospital course, adult respiratory distress syndrome and pneumonia can further complicate the picture.

Mechanical ventilation is appropriate in patients who suffer from hypoxemic or hypercapneic respiratory failure. In patients who are endotracheally intubated, positive end-expiratory pressure should be used as a tactic to recruit alveoli, raise mean airway pressures, and decrease shunt. Continuous positive airway pressure or pressure support should also be added to improve compliance and decrease shunt.[54] There is no single mode of ventilation that has been found to be best for patients with flail chest or pulmonary contusion.[32]

Often, patients with significant chest wall injury with impending respiratory failure are successfully managed without an endotracheal tube. There is some evidence that noninvasive ventilation (NIV) strategies, such as mask-delivered continuous positive airway pressure, may decrease mortality, nosocomial infections,[55,56] and ventilator days.[55] Ferrer and colleagues[57] and Hernandez and colleagues[58] have shown that NIV positive pressure ventilation compared with high-flow nasal cannula oxygen alone can avoid or significantly delay intubation in critically ill patients. Of course, NIV should not be attempted in the patient who is in shock, profoundly hypoxemic, or acidotic. Patients should be monitored in the intensive care unit, where endotracheal intubation may be expeditiously performed if necessary. It is prudent to have a predetermined threshold for hypoxemia or acidosis, below which intubation and mechanical ventilation are indicated. Although there is no well-studied time limit for how long one should persist with a trial of NIV, 1 to 4 hours seems reasonable if the patient remains hemodynamically stable, is able to clear secretions, and oxygenation remains adequate. If there is no improvement seen in this time frame, the patient should be intubated and placed on mechanical ventilation.[59] The clinician should also remember that trauma patients, particularly those with severe head injury or significant bleeding risk, generally require a higher arterial oxygen level than other critically ill populations.

Surgical Management

Despite the increasing popularity of SSRF, this operation is performed in less than 1% of patients with flail chest. Lack of widespread adoption of SSRF is likely caused by unfamiliarity with the technique, lack of subspecialty ownership (ie, trauma, orthopedic, and thoracic surgery), and a perceived lack of evidence-based indications.[60]

Several prospective studies, including three randomized trials[21–23] and two meta-analyses,[61,62] have documented substantial benefit to SSRF for the specific indication of flail chest. Outcomes analyzed consistently were respiratory failure, pneumonia, tracheostomy, and mortality. Additional outcomes, such as narcotic requirements, pulmonary function testing, and long-term functional outcomes, have not been well studied, although some preliminary data exist documenting benefit.[22,63,64]

One limitation to the aforementioned literature involves the tremendous clinical and radiographic variability of patients with flail chest. Injuries may range from unicortical, nondisplaced fractures in stable patients to severely displaced fractures with substantial volume loss in intubated, critically ill patients with multiple competing injuries. This variability in disease severity may account for recent negative studies of SSRF.[65] Further research is needed to identify specific patients with flail chest who will benefit most from SSRF. However, the preponderance of data in this patient population suggest a lasting benefit to SSRF.

The benefit of SSRF in non–flail chest fracture patterns has also been evaluated, the most common being multiple severely (bicortical) displaced fractures.[24,64] Also, patients with less impressive radiographic fracture patterns (eg, nondisplaced or minimally displaced fractures) may rarely present with refractory pain or respiratory compromise. One such example is a patient with localized, exquisite pain with respiration over one or two fractures, accompanied by a painful "clicking" sensation with palpation. Although there have been anecdotal reports of marked symptomatic improving following SSRF in such cases, nothing has been published.

Traditional contraindications to SSRF include pulmonary contusion and severe traumatic brain injury. Severe pulmonary contusions may drive acute respiratory outcomes to a greater extent than rib fractures. However, it is unclear to what degree this phenomenon exists in patients with mild to moderate contusions. Although Voggenreiter and colleagues[66] reported poor outcomes in a group of 10 patients with pulmonary contusion (diagnosed by CXR) who underwent SSRF, most of these patients underwent SSRF either on retreat following emergency throracotomy or greater than 7 days from injury. The efficacy of SSRF in patients with traumatic brain injury also remains to be studied specifically; most studies of SSRF exclude these patients. Early clinical and radiographic risk stratification of these patients have poor predictive ability.

Debate continues as to the optimal timing of SSRF. The operation has traditionally been considered a salvage maneuver that should be reserved for patients who have failed a trial of maximal nonoperative management. This trial period ranged from 7 to 14 days. However, there has been a recent paradigm shift among proponents of SSRF toward earlier intervention, the logic being that the (often) predictable deterioration observed among patients with severe chest wall injuries managed nonoperatively may be avoided by early SSRF. To this end, most modern series of SSRF have performed the operation within 72 hours of injury, and ideally within 24 hours of injury.[61,64,65,67] Additional advantages to early operation include less inflammation and callous formation, and an early opportunity to evacuate the pleural space and place directed analgesic catheters.

Patients being considered for SSRF should undergo CT chest with three-dimensional reconstruction if available (**Fig. 1**) to assist with fracture identification, selection of fractures for fixation, and assessment of the pleural space. Surgery should be performed on resuscitated patients without competing, serious injuries (ie, unstable spine fractures and uncontrolled intracranial pressures). In general, ribs 1, 2, 11, and 12 should not be repaired because of minimal contribution to chest wall integrity and difficulty of exposure. Fractures of ribs 3 to 10 should be considered for repair, and both fracture lines should be stabilized in the case of flail chest.[68] Fractures within 2.5 cm of the transverse process posteriorly should not be repaired because there is rarely adequate bone length on the posterior fracture fragment to secure either a plate or intramedullary strut. Very anterior fractures require fixation to either cartilage or sternum. These advanced techniques have been described but represent off-label uses of current Food and Drug Administration–approved fixation systems.

Although percutaneous and thoracoscopic techniques of SSRF have been described,[69] the most commonly used approach remains open thoracotomy. However, modern techniques of minimally invasive, open SSRF have eliminated virtually all muscle division, and the notion that SSRF should be avoided secondary to incisional

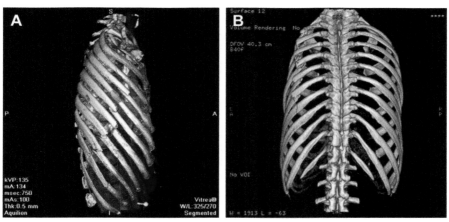

Fig. 1. (*A, B*) Three-dimensional computed tomography reconstructions of severe flail chest. (*Courtesy of* Dr Thomas White, Murray, UT; and Drs Cornelius Dyke and Steven Briggs, Fargo, ND.)

pain is no longer valid.[68,70] Muscle-sparing SSRF involves a shift away from traditional thoracic incisions, which are designed to provide exposure to intrapleural structures (and thus mirror the course of the ribs), to SSRF-specific exposures (**Fig. 2**), which are designed to expose multiple ribs without dividing muscle. Newer equipment, including right-angled drilling and screw driving systems, has greatly facilitated repair of rib fractures beneath overlying, intact myocutaneous flaps.

Anterior fracture series may be exposed with the patient in the supine position, and through an oblique incision along the inframammary fold. A subpectoral flap is then developed, which provides excellent exposure to anterior ribs 4 to 6. Anterior fractures of the third rib may be approached through a small horizontal incision directly over the fracture, with splitting of the fibers of the pectoralis major and minor muscles.

Lateral fracture series may be approached with the patient in the lateral decubitus position, and

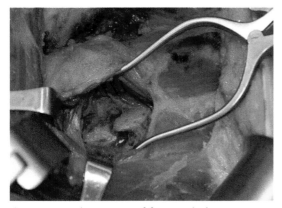

Fig. 2. Surgical exposure of fractured rib.

through a 7-to-9-cm longitudinal incision, placed along the anterior border of the latissimus dorsi muscle. The anterior border is then developed, and a flap is raised underneath the muscle such that it may be retracted posteriorly. This exposes the muscle branches of the serratus anterior, which may be split to expose the rib fractures. Care must be taken at this point to avoid injury to the long thoracic nerve.

Posterior fractures are typically the most difficult to repair because of proximity to the transverse process, angulation of the rib, and subscapular location. These fractures may be approached with the patient in the prone position and the ipsilateral arm supported on a table that is lowered approximately eight inches relative to the operating table. This maneuver allows for 4 to 8 inches of lateralization of the scapula and facilitates exposure of posterior, subscapular fractures. A longitudinal incision is then made just medial to the scapular tip, and the triangle of auscultation is developed.

Patients with multiple fracture series (flail chest) typically have a combination of either anterior and lateral fractures, or lateral and posterior fractures. Either fracture pattern may be approached through two of the incisions described previously. Alternatively, a traditional posterolateral thoracotomy may be used. Another common fracture pattern is an anterior flail chest; that is, bilateral anterior fractures series. This fracture pattern may be effectively exposed via bilateral inframammary incisions.

Fractures may be stabilized using suture, intramedullary struts, or plates (**Figs. 3** and **4**). Plates may be permanent or absorbable, although only the former is currently Food and Drug Administration–approved for use in rib repair. By far the most

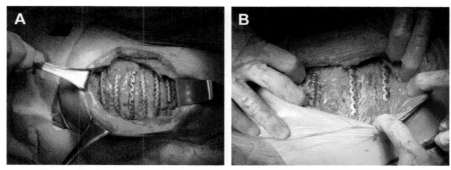

Fig. 3. (*A, B*) In situ surgical rib fixation. (*Courtesy of* Dr Thomas White, Murray, UT; and Drs Cornelius Dyke and Steven Briggs, Fargo, ND.)

experience in rib fixation has been with the use of permanent plates, and an important technical advancement in SSRF has been the creation of low-profile, titanium, rib-specific plates that mimic the contour and elasticity of native ribs (see **Fig. 3**). Although there are no strong data to support the use of plates over struts, there has been some

concern regarding the structural integrity of the latter.[71] Fixation should aim to immobilize the fracture enough to allow pain relief and healing, but leave room for micromovement at the fracture site to promote osteoclast activity and callous formation. This balance may be achieved by avoiding "overtightening" the screws on the plate.

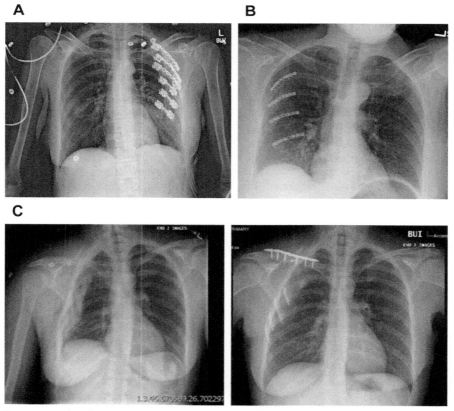

Fig. 4. (*A, B*) Postoperative chest radiographs after surgical rib fixation. (*C*) Preoperative and postoperative chest radiographs of same patient showing severe volume loss/deformity and restoration of thoracic cage. (*Courtesy of* Dr Brian Kim, Springfield, MO; and Dr Thomas White, Murray, UT.)

Sternal Fractures

The sternum consists of the manubrium, body, and xiphoid process, and rests directly anterior to the right ventricle, pulmonary trunk, and ascending aorta. Fracture of the sternum should thus alert the clinician to the possibility of injury to the underlying mediastinal structures, particularly blunt cardiac injury. The incidence of sternal fractures has decreased markedly since the widespread adoption of driver and passenger side airbags. Fractures typically occur at either the angle or body of the sternum, and are manifest by chest pain, tenderness, and, rarely, instability. Both anteroposterior and lateral CXRs are usually inadequate to diagnose and fully characterize sternal fractures; CT chest is warranted when the diagnosis is suspected clinically.

Most sternal fractures may be managed successfully using a nonoperative approach centered on analgesia, physical therapy, and exclusion of underlying intrathoracic injuries. There are a paucity of data to inform objective indications for operative repair. However, repair has traditionally been considered in cases of severe displacement and/or deformity (see **Fig. 4**), loss of sternal continuity, and intractable pain.

Sternal repair was first undertaken in 1943 using a Kirschner wire.[72] Since then, permanent plates have become the standard fixation modality,[73] although absorbable plates have also been used.[74] The surgical technique consists of a midline, longitudinal incision centered over the fractures, with exposure of the fracture, evacuation of the surrounding hematoma, and debridement of nonviable tissue. Reduction forceps are then introduced laterally into the surrounding intercostal spaces, being careful to avoid injury to the internal thoracic vessels. Bicortical fixation is recommended, with screw length estimated by CT and intraoperative calibration.

REFERENCES

1. Available at: http://hcupnet.ahrq.gov/HCUPnet.jsp. Accessed June 14, 2016.
2. Bulger EM, Arneson MA, Mock CN, et al. Rib fractures in the elderly. J Trauma 2000;48:1040–7.
3. Flagel BT, Luchette FA, Reed RL, et al. Half a dozen ribs: the breakpoint for mortality. Surgery 2005;138:717–25.
4. Holcomb JB, McMullin NR, Kozar RA, et al. Morbidity from rib fractures increases after age 45. J Am Coll Surg 2003;196:549–55.
5. Sharma OP, Oswanski MF, Jolly S, et al. Perils of rib fractures. Am Surg 2008;74:310–4.
6. Dehghan N, deMestral C, McKee MD, et al. Flail chest injuries: a review of outcomes and treatment practices from the National Trauma Data Bank. J Trauma Acute Care Surg 2014;76:462–8.
7. Kerr-Valentic MA, Arthur M, Mullins RJ, et al. Rib fracture pain and disability: can we do better? J Trauma 2003;54:1058–63.
8. Landercasper J, Cogbill TH, Lindesmith LA. Long-term disability after flail chest injury. J Trauma 1984;24:410–4.
9. Beal SL, Oreskovich MR. Long-term disability associated with flail chest injury. Am J Surg 1985;150:324–6.
10. Fabricant L, Ham B, Mullins R, et al. Prolonged pain and disability are common after rib fractures. Am J Surg 2013;205:511–5.
11. Clark GC, Schecter WP, Trunkey DD. Variables affecting outcome in blunt chest trauma: flail chest versus pulmonary contusion. J Trauma 1988;28:298–304.
12. Richardson JD, Adams L, Flint LM. Selective management of flail chest and pulmonary contusion. Ann Surg 1982;196:481–7.
13. Breasted J. The Edwin Smith surgical papyrus. Chicago: Chicago University Press; 1980.
14. Hagen K. Multiple rib fractures treated with a drinker respirator: a case report. J Bone Joint Surg Am 1945;27:330–4.
15. Cohen EA. Treatment of the flail chest by towel clip traction. Am J Surg 1955;90:517–21.
16. Avery EE, Benson DW, Morch ET. Critically crushed chests: a new method of treatment with continuous mechanical hyperventilation to produce alkalotic apnea and internal pneumatic stabilization. J Thorac Surg 1956;32:291–311.
17. Dor J, Chasson J, Paoli JM, et al. Treatment of traumatic thoracic "shutters" by "internal pneumatic stabilization". Am Chir Thorac Cardiovasc 1964;3:314–22.
18. Trinkel JK, Richardson JD, Franz JL, et al. Management of flail chest without mechanical ventilation. Ann Thorac Surg 1975;19:355–63.
19. Shackford SR, Smith DE, Zarins CK, et al. The management of flail chest. A comparison of ventilatory and non-ventilatory treatment. Am J Surg 1976;132:759–62.
20. Bemelman M, Poeze M, Blokhuis TJ, et al. Historic overview of treatment techniques for rib fractures and flail chest. Eur J Trauma Emerg Surg 2010;36:407–15.
21. Tanaka H, Yukioka T, Yamaguti Y, et al. Surgical stabilization of internal pneumatic stabilization? A prospective randomized study of management of severe flail chest patients. J Trauma 2002;52(4):727–32 [discussion: 732].
22. Granetzny AM, Abd El-Aal M, Emam E, et al. Surgical versus conservative treatment of flail chest.

Evaluation of the pulmonary status. Interact Cardiovasc Thorac Surg 2005;4(6):583–7.

23. Marasco SF, Davies AR, Cooper J, et al. Prospective, randomized controlled trial of operative rib fixation in traumatic flail chest. J Am Coll Surg 2013; 216(5):924–32.

24. Pieracci FM, Lin Y, Rodi M, et al. A prospective, controlled clinical evaluation of surgical stabilization of severe rib fractures. J Trauma Acute Care Surg 2016;80(2):187–94.

25. Wilson RF, Murray C, Antonenko DR. Nonpenetrating thoracic injuries. Surg Clin North Am 1977;57:17–36.

26. Shorr RM, Crittenden M, Indeck M, et al. Blunt thoracic trauma. Analysis of 515 patients. Ann Surg 1987;206:200–5.

27. Shweiki E, Klena J, Wood GC, et al. Assessing the true risk of abdominal solid organ injury in hospitalized rib fracture patients. J Trauma 2001;50:684–8.

28. Livingston D, Lavery R, Passannante M, et al. Admission or observation is not necessary after a negative abdominal computed tomographic scan in patients with suspected blunt abdominal trauma: results of a prospective, multi-institutional trial. J Trauma 1998;44:273–80.

29. Cameron P, Dziukas L, Hadj A, et al. Rib fractures in major trauma. Aust N Z J Surg 1996;66:530–4.

30. Garcia VF, Gotschall CS, Eichelberger MR, et al. Rib fractures in children: a marker of severe trauma. J Trauma 1990;30:695–700.

31. American College of Surgeons Committee on Trauma. Advanced trauma life support. 9th edition. Chicago: American College of Surgeons; 2014.

32. Simon B, Ebert J, Bokhari F, et al. Management of pulmonary contusion and flail chest: an eastern association for the surgery of trauma practice management guideline. J Trauma Acute Care Surg 2012;73: s351–61.

33. Livingston DH, Shogan B, John P, et al. CT diagnosis of rib fractures and prediction of acute respiratory failure. J Trauma 2008;64:905–11.

34. Brink M, Deunk J, Dekker HM, et al. Criteria for the selective use of chest computed tomography in blunt trauma patients. Eur Radiol 2010;20:818–28.

35. Rodriguez RM, Anglin D, Langdorf MI, et al. Validation of a decision instrument for selective chest imaging in blunt trauma. JAMA Surg 2013;148: 940–6.

36. Unsworth A, Curtis K, Asha SE. Treatments for blunt chest trauma and their impact on patient outcomes and health service delivery. Scand J Trauma Resusc Emerg Med 2015;23:17.

37. Sahr SM, Webb ML, Renner CH, et al. Implementation of a rib fracture triage protocol in elderly trauma patients. J Trauma Nurs 2013;20:172–5.

38. Todd SR, McNally MM, Holcomb JB, et al. A multidisciplinary clinical pathway decreases rib fracture-associated infectious morbidity and mortality in high-risk trauma patients. Am J Surg 2006;192:806–11.

39. Menditto VG, Gabrielli B, Marcosignori M, et al. A management of blunt thoracic trauma in an emergency department observation unit: a pre-post observational study. J Trauma Acute Care Surg 2012;72:222–8.

40. Moon MR, Luchette FA, Gibson SW, et al. Prospective randomized comparison of epidural versus parenteral opioid analgesia in thoracic trauma. Ann Surg 1999;229:684–91.

41. Wu CL, Jani ND, Perkins FM, et al. Thoracic epidural analgesia versus intravenous patient-controlled analgesia for the treatment of rib fracture pain after motor vehicle crash. J Trauma 1999;47:564–7.

42. Ingalls NK, Horton ZA, Bettendorf M, et al. Randomized, double-blind, placebo controlled trial using lidocaine patch 5% in traumatic rib fractures. J Am Coll Surg 2010;210:205–9.

43. Zink KA, Mayberry JC, Peck EG, et al. Lidocaine patches reduce pain in patients with rib fractures. Am Surg 2011;77:438–42.

44. Gage A, Rivara F, Wang J, et al. The effect of epidural placement in patients after blunt thoracic trauma. J Trauma Acute Care Surg 2014;76:39–46.

45. Wisner DH. A stepwise logistic regression analysis of factors affecting morbidity and mortality after thoracic trauma: effect of epidural anesthesia. J Trauma 1990;30:799–804.

46. Hashemzadeh S, Hashemzadeh K, Hosseinzadeh H, et al. Comparison thoracic epidural and intercostal block to improve ventilation parameters and reduce pain in patients with multiple rib fractures. J Cardiovasc Thorac Res 2011;3:87–91.

47. Mackersie RC, Karagianes TG, Hoyt DB, et al. Prospective evaluation of epidural and intravenous administration of fentanyl for pain control and restoration of ventilatory function following multiple rib fractures. J Trauma 1991;31:449–51.

48. Bulger EM, Edwards T, Klotz P, et al. Epidural analgesia improves outcome after multiple rib fractures. Surgery 2004;136:426–30.

49. Zaw AA, Murry J, Hoang D, Chen K, et al. Epidural anesthesia after rib fractures. Am Surg 2015;81: 950–4.

50. Auroy Y, Narchi P, Messiah A, et al. Serious complications related to regional anesthesia: results of a prospective survey in France. Anesthesiology 1997;87:479–86.

51. Ahn Y, Gohrlinger K, Alam HB, et al. Pain-associated respiratory failure in chest trauma. Anesthesiology 2013;118:701–8.

52. Britt T, Sturm R, Ricardi R, et al. Comparative evaluation of continuous intercostal nerve block or epidural analgesia on the rate of respiratory complications, intensive care unit, and hospital stay

following traumatic rib fractures: a retrospective review. Local Reg Anesth 2015;8:79–84.

53. Truitt MS, Murry J, Amos J, et al. Continuous intercostal nerve blockade for rib fractures: ready for prime time? J Trauma 2011;71:1548–52.

54. Schweiger JW, Downs JB, Smith RA. Chest wall disruption with and without acute lung injury: effects of continuous positive airway pressure therapy on ventilation and perfusion relationships. Crit Care Med 2003;31:2364–70.

55. Gunduz M, Unlugenc H, Ozalevli M, et al. A comparative study of continuous positive airway pressure (CPAP) and intermittent positive pressure ventilation (IPPV) in patients with flail chest. Emerg Med J 2005;22:325–9.

56. Tanaka H, Tajimi K, Endoh Y, et al. Pneumatic stabilization for flail chest injury: an 11 year study. Surg Today 2001;31:12–7.

57. Ferrer M, Esquinas A, Leon M, et al. Noninvasive ventilation in severe hypoxemic respiratory failure: a randomized clinical trial. Am J Respir Crit Care Med 2003;168:1438–44.

58. Hernandez G, Fernandez R, Lopez-Reina P, et al. Noninvasive ventilation reduces intubation in chest trauma-related hypoxemia: a randomized clinical trial. Chest 2010;137:74–80.

59. Karcz MK, Papadakos PJ. Noninvasive ventilation in trauma. World J Crit Care Med 2015;4:47–54.

60. Mayberry JC, Ham LB, Schipper PH, et al. Surveyed opinion of American trauma, orthopedic, and thoracic surgeons on rib and sternal fracture repair. J Trauma 2009;66(3):875–9.

61. Leinicke JA, Elmore L, Freeman BD, et al. Operative management of rib fractures in the setting of flail chest: a systematic review and meta-analysis. Ann Surg 2013;258(6):914–21.

62. Slobogean GP, MacPherson CA, Sun T, et al. Surgical fixation vs nonoperative management of flail chest: a meta-analysis. J Am Coll Surg 2013; 216(2):302–11.e1.

63. Majercik S, Cannon Q, Granger SR, et al. Long-term patient outcomes after surgical stabilization of rib fractures. Am J Surg 2014;208(1):88–92.

64. Doben AR, Eriksson EA, Denlinger CE, et al. Surgical rib fixation for flail chest deformity improves liberation from mechanical ventilation. J Crit Care 2014; 29(1):139–43.

65. DeFreest L, Tafen M, Bhakta A, et al. Open reduction and internal fixation of rib fractures in polytrauma patients with flail chest. Am J Surg 2016;211(4):761–7.

66. Voggenreiter G, Neudeck F, Aufmkolk M, et al. Operative chest wall stabilization in flail chest: outcomes of patients with or without pulmonary contusion. J Am Coll Surg 1998;187(2):130–8.

67. Pieracci FM, Rodil M, Stovall RT, et al. Surgical stabilization of severe rib fractures. J Trauma Acute Care Surg 2015;78(4):883–7.

68. Marasco S, Liew S, Edwards E, et al. Analysis of bone healing in flail chest injury: do we need to fix both fractures per rib? J Trauma Acute Care Surg 2014;77(3):452–8.

69. Pieracci FM, Johnson J, Stoval RT, et al. Completely thoracoscopic, intra-pleural reduction and fixation of severe rib fractures. Trauma Case Reports 2015;1: 39–43.

70. Hasenboehler EA, Bernard AC, Bottiggi AJ, et al. Treatment of traumatic flail chest with muscular sparing open reduction and internal fixation: description of a surgical technique. J Trauma 2011;71(2):494–501.

71. Marasco SF, Liovic P, Sutalo ID. Structural integrity of intramedullary rib fixation using a single bioresorbable screw. J Trauma Acute Care Surg 2012; 73(3):668–73.

72. McKim LH. A method of fixation for fractures of the sternum. Ann Surg 1943;118:168–80.

73. Ergene G, Tulay CM, Anasiz H. Sternal fixation with nonspecific plate. Ann Thorac Cardiovasc Surg 2013;19(5):364–7.

74. Ahmad K, Katballe N, Pilegaard H. Fixation of sternal fracture using absorbable plating system, three years follow-up. J Thorac Dis 2015;7(5):E131–4.

Minimal Invasive Repair of Pectus Excavatum and Carinatum

Hans Pilegaard, MD[a,b],*, Peter Bjørn Licht, MD, PhD[c]

KEYWORDS

- Chest wall deformity • Pectus excavatum • Pectus carinatum • Minimally invasive surgery
- Thoracoscopy

KEY POINTS

- Chest wall anomalies almost exclusively consist of pectus excavatum and pectus carinatum.
- With increased awareness on the Internet, the number of patients who seek help continues to rise, primarily for cosmetic reasons.
- Minimally invasive surgery has become the gold standard for surgical repair of pectus excavatum.
- Open reconstruction has been the standard approach for surgical treatment, but over the past decade, surgery has largely been replaced by compression techniques that use a brace, and cosmetic results are good.
- Rare combinations of pectus excavatum and carinatum may be treated by newer surgical methods.

INTRODUCTION

Chest wall anomalies almost exclusively consist of pectus excavatum and pectus carinatum. Pectus excavatum is the most frequent form (except in South America) and represents approximately 90% of all chest wall anomalies. Historical reviews[1,2] mention that it was first depicted in 1510 by Leonardo da Vinci,[3] first described as a disease entity in 1594 by Bauhinus,[4] and the first attempt to correct pectus excavatum was performed by the German surgeon Ludwig Meyer in 1911.[5]

The modern era of surgical correcting of chest anomalies started when Ravitch published his article in 1949.[6] Initially, his operation included total resection of the involved cartilages as well as parts of the ribs, but it was later modified to preserve the perichondrium, which allowed new cartilage formation. Several modifications have since been introduced in the literature and the open approach was the gold standard for chest wall corrections during the following 50 years. In 1998, Nuss and colleagues[7] published the first paper on minimal invasive repair of pectus excavatum, which soon changed surgical correction in general and his approach is now considered the gold standard for correction of pectus excavatum. Most likely, this concept of minimally invasive surgery also fueled development of new minimal invasive techniques for correction of pectus carinatum.

PECTUS EXCAVATUM

This is the most frequent chest wall anomaly, which is seen 4 to 6 times more often in male compared with female individuals. The incidence varies geographically and affects approximately 1:3 to 400 male individuals in the Western world.[8]

[a] Department of Clinical Medicine, Aarhus University, 99 Palle Juul-Jensens Boulevard, Aarhus N DK-8200, Denmark; [b] Department of Cardiothoracic and Vascular Surgery, Aarhus University Hospital Skejby, 99 Palle Juul-Jensens Boulevard, Aarhus N DK-8200, Denmark; [c] Department of Cardiothoracic Surgery, Odense University Hospital, 29 Søndre Boulevard, Odense DK-5000, Denmark
* Corresponding author. Department of Clinical Medicine, Aarhus University, 99 Palle Juul-Jensens Boulevard, Aarhus N DK-8200, Denmark.
E-mail address: pilegaard@dadlnet.dk

Thorac Surg Clin 27 (2017) 123–131
http://dx.doi.org/10.1016/j.thorsurg.2017.01.005
1547-4127/17/© 2017 Elsevier Inc. All rights reserved.

Previously, pectus excavatum was considered only a cosmetic problem for the patients, but recent studies have shown that cardiac performance may be reduced up to 20% and chest mobility also may be reduced.[9–12]

Following the introduction of a minimal invasive surgical correction technique and an increased awareness by fast dissemination on the Internet, the number of patients who seek advice for surgery has increased considerably in the past decade.

Patient Selection

Most patients seek correction for cosmetic reasons[13] and are less concerned with any concomitant reduction in cardiac performance, but more than 60% of these patients actually report cardiopulmonary symptoms when asked.[14] We believe that surgery for cosmetic reasons is a good indication, because studies show significant improvements in quality of life after surgical correction.[12,15] It is also a good indication to operate patients who present with symptoms from reduced cardiac performance, which is thought to result from compression of the heart as well as reduced movements of the chest.[9,16,17]

Many surgeons have used the Haller index as a discriminator for surgical correction. This is based on a computed tomography (CT) scan of the chest and represents the ratio between the transverse and the anterior-posterior diameter of the chest, in which a value of 3.2 to 3.25 was set as an indication for surgery.[18] We believe the Haller index is a poor measure to guide patients and surgeons, because abnormal values may be found in normal chest shapes and some patients are severely affected psychologically and cosmetically by their chest wall anomaly even when the Haller index is lower than 3.2. In addition, the Haller index is not correlated to the physiologic symptoms of a pectus excavatum.[19]

The optimal age for surgical correction of pectus excavatum is controversial. Most surgeons prefer to operate patients in the beginning of puberty, when the growth spurt starts. It is an advantage to postpone surgery in female individuals until they have a good demarcation of their breast, because that allows for the surgical incisions to be hidden in the inframammary fold. In Asia, many patients undergo surgical correction when they are much younger, as young as 2 to 6 years,[20] but many Western surgeons discourage this practice for ethical reasons. They argue that most likely very young patients are not aware of their pectus excavatum and less so concerned about their chest wall deformity. Furthermore, they may have

difficulty understanding the impact of surgical treatment and the restrictions that follow. Finally, Nuss observed a higher risk of recurrence if the pectus bar was removed before puberty.[21] An upper limit for surgical correction is not yet been defined. When the Nuss technique was published, it was not considered feasible to operate adults, but with the increasing experience this has not been a major problem and patients older than 70 years have been surgically corrected.[22]

Preoperative Assessment

In most patients, their history combined with a thorough clinical examination and a simple chest radiograph are enough to make the decision for surgical correction. In some health care systems, and particularly when private insurance is involved, more thorough assessments may be required, including chest CT scan, lung function tests, and echocardiography, but we only consider these necessary if there is clinical suspicion of comorbidity, such as Marfan syndrome.

Surgical Technique

Preparation and positioning

Immediately before surgery an epidural catheter should be inserted, which also allows for optimal pain management postoperatively. The operation is performed with general anesthesia, and the patient is placed in the supine position on the far right side of the operating table, which allows for optimum free movement of the thoracoscope during the procedure (**Fig. 1**). The patient's right arm or even both arms should be abducted and extended to the front of the head (**Fig. 2**). Prophylactic antibiotics are mandatory and should be given intravenously and continued for 1 to 3 days depending on local tradition.

Surgical approach

First, the deepest point of the pectus excavatum is identified because the best result is achieved when this point is lifted (**Fig. 3**). Rarely, this point is not the ideal and the sternum is raised too much, in which case the bar needs to be reinserted more obliquely. The points in which the bar should enter and exit the chest wall are then marked on the skin. Very importantly, they are different from the skin incisions, which are always lateral, and should be just medial to the highest point of the pectus excavatum (**Fig. 4**). The correct spot may be tested by pressing a finger on the skin from the outside while viewing the thoracoscopic monitor to see that this point is in line with the deepest area of the pectus excavatum. We use a thoracoscope only in the right chest, but some surgeons prefer to view

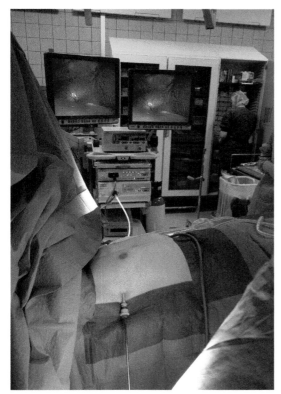

Fig. 1. The patient is placed in the supine position on the far right side of the operating table, which allows for optimum free movement of the thoracoscope during the procedure.

both sides of the chest during the procedure, and the level of insertion depends on personal preferences. Nuss inserted the thoracoscope in the lower part of the chest wall,[23] which we consider less optimal because it introduces a potential risk of penetrating the diaphragm. More importantly, we believe it decreases the caudal view inside the chest cavity, and we therefore prefer to have the

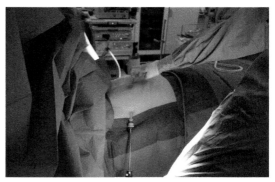

Fig. 3. The deepest point of the pectus excavatum is identified because the best result is achieved when this point is lifted.

trocar at the level of the nipple, which allows full view of the chest without restrictions.

A tunnel under the sternum is created with a dedicated "introducer" (**Fig. 5**). It is very important that the tip of the introducer keeps a close contact with the backside of the sternum to avoid injury to the pericardium or the heart. If the patient's pectus excavation is extremely deep, there are various methods to facilitate the preparation of this tunnel while decreasing the risk of injury. One may use a crane to lift the sternum,[24] or the assistant may simply lift the sternum with 2 retractors through the incisions prepared for the bar while the tunnel is prepared.[25] Likewise, a vacuum bell that covers the deepest point of the excavation may be used to lift the sternum.[26] In patients with severe or extreme pectus excavatum, it is most often required to use more than 1 pectus bar and subsequently also more than 1 introducer to lift the sternum. As many as 3 pectus bars may be required in extreme situations (**Fig. 6**). When this is required,

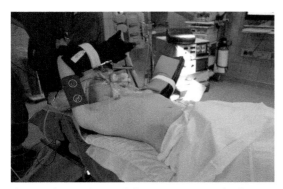

Fig. 2. The patient's right arm or even both arms should be abducted and extended to the front of the head.

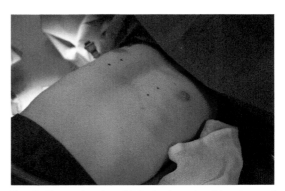

Fig. 4. The points in which the bar should enter and exit the chest wall are marked on the skin. They are different from the skin incisions, which are always lateral, and they should be just medial to the highest point of the pectus excavatum.

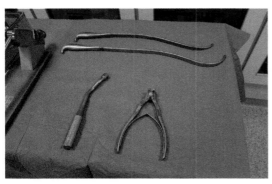

Fig. 5. Special surgical tools are needed for minimally invasive correction of pectus excavatum. In the top, there are 2 dedicated "introducers" that are used to create a tunnel under the sternum.

we recommend placing the first introducer more cranial than the deepest point, which may then be elevated 3 to 4 cm, allowing for an easier and safer pass of the second introducer.

The thoracoscope in the right chest is used to view the safe guiding of the introducer below the sternum. When the introducer has passed the deepest point of the excavatum, some surgeons prefer to insert the thoracoscope in the left chest to view the final passing of the introducer, but we do not think this is necessary. CO_2 insufflation may improve the view inside the chest cavity, but for most experienced surgeons this does not add any benefits. A special rigid thoracoscope named a "pectoscope" was developed by Park[28] to assist during preparation of the tunnel below the sternum, but it is not essential if it is elevated by one of the "crane" techniques mentioned.

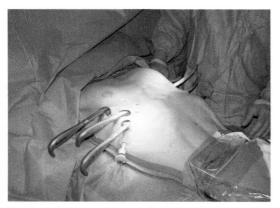

Fig. 6. As many as 3 pectus bars may be required in extreme situations, in which case we recommend to place the first introducer cranial to the deepest point, which may then be elevated 3 to 4 cm allowing for an easier and safer pass of the second introducer.

In his original article, Nuss and colleagues[7] describe that the bar length should be measured from one midaxillary line to the other, but earlier this caused a problem of bar flipping in 15% of the patients. We use a shorter bar, typically 2 to 3 inches shorter, because it reduces the risk of bar flipping.[27] Nuss[18] later introduced a lateral stabilizer that was fixated and he used additional sutures at the opposite end of the bar, which reduced the risk of flipping to approximately 1%, which is comparable with the shorter bar technique. In most patients, the fixation is on the left side of the patient because in the very rare situation that the end of the pectus bar without stabilizer drops into the chest, this part will not compress or injure the heart on the right side. In addition, to further prevent the bar from dropping into the chest, the shorter bar is placed asymmetrically on the chest wall so that the end that does not have the stabilizer also covers 2 ribs. The stabilizer is placed at the very end of the pectus bar where it lies flat on the chest wall very close to the exit point from the chest cavity. A steel wire is used to anchor the stabilizer to the bar but it is not necessary to fixate it to the rib, which would also make it more difficult to remove the bar and stabilizer at a later stage. Other surgeons prefer to fix the bar to the rib with multiple sutures and fiber wires, and use 2 stabilizers or use a "claw fixator," a specially designed fixator, which hooks the rib and is fixed to the bar.[28] If the exit and entrance points into the chest are not medial to the highest points of the pectus deformity, there is a risk of "stripping," which means that the intercostal muscle detaches from the rib because the forces from the bar are transferred to the intercostal muscle when there is no support from the ribs. However, adding a stabilizer or a suture that connects the 2 adjacent ribs can solve this problem. Park and colleagues[29] use a different technique, because they penetrate the chest wall laterally and therefore require a special support for the bar, a hinge point, which is fixed to the ribs.

Immediate Postoperative Care

Air is inevitably introduced into the chest cavity during surgery and is evacuated by a simple chest drain under water seal while the anesthesiologist inflates the lung using positive airway pressure, but the chest drain is removed immediately thereafter and under normal circumstances a chest tube is not required after surgery. The patient is extubated in the operating room and it is usually sufficient to observe the patient in a recovery area for 1 to 2 hours before he or she returns to the normal ward. All patients are mobilized in the evening on the same day of surgery and are encouraged to walk frequently the following days. In our institution, 85% of patients can be discharged from the hospital on the second postoperative day and very few patients are hospitalized more than 4 days.

Pain management is extremely important and begins with an epidural catheter preoperatively. Following surgery, in the recovery room, it is important to confirm that pain management is sufficient before the patient is transferred back to the normal ward. Additional oral analgesics are started on the day of surgery in the evening and vary with local tradition. For years, our patients have been satisfied with a standard regimen of paracetamol 1 g × 4 for 4 to 5 weeks in combination with ibuprofen 400 mg × 3 for 3 to 4 weeks. On postoperative day 1, we start opioids, typically oxycodone 10 to 20 mg twice a day depending on body weight for 2 weeks, and the epidural is terminated on the second postoperative day. On the second postoperative, day we get a chest radiograph with both anterior-posterior and lateral projections to verify that the pectus bar is in the correct position before scheduled discharge on postoperative day 3.[30]

Rehabilitation and Recovery

After discharge from the hospital, the patients have several restrictions for the first 6 weeks. They should not carry heavy weights exceeding 2 kg in front of the body or 5 kg on the back. They should not engage in sports activity or bicycle riding, and they should restrain from twisting of the upper body. It is frequently a problem for patients to sleep because of pain and they are allowed to sleep only in the supine position to avoid bar dislocation. In addition, sleeping on the sides or on the abdominal side is very painful just after correction, but this pain gradually ceases over the next 5 to 7 weeks, allowing a more habitual sleeping position.

The patients should be encouraged to walk at least twice every day and follow simple muscle exercises as suggested by the physiotherapist. Six weeks after discharge, all patients are seen in the outpatient clinic in the hospital for clinical evaluation and a chest radiograph. If everything appears in order, they are advised to begin swimming, slow jogging, or bicycling, and only gradually increase their activity to their preoperative level over the subsequent 6 weeks. During the entire period in which the bar(s) are in situ, the patients should avoid heavy contact sports. Typically, this period extends for 3 years, after which the patient returns for pectus bar removal; patients should be encouraged to contact the hospital earlier if they experience any problems with the pectus bar, but this almost never occurs.

Clinical Results

Most patients are very satisfied with the cosmetic result after minimal invasive repair of pectus excavatum, and less than 5% are dissatisfied.[21] Cardiac performance also increases approximately 25% after correction in children and adolescents,[17] and the maximum oxygen uptake in adults also increases significantly, at least after open correction.[31]

In experienced hands, complications are rare but mortality has been published.[32] We have performed more than 1700 consecutive procedures without any mortality. Deep wound infection occurred in 1% but was treated conservatively with antibiotics without removal of the bar system in almost all patients. Even if the pectus bar is visible through the skin defect, the patient may be treated successfully without bar removal by vacuum-assisted closure of the defect in combination with antibiotics. After pectus bar removal, after 3 years the recurrence rate is less than 1% and very few develop a pectus carinatum, which may be corrected by external compression if it does not regress spontaneously following bar removal.

The Nuss technique also may be used in previous failed open procedures even though the chest wall often developed rigidity due to ossification of the new cartilage is these patients.

Vacuum Bell Treatment

Vacuum bell treatment is a new noninvasive treatment that may be used if patients refuse surgery or in young children with a very small pectus excavatum. Generally, it will not correct their pectus excavatum completely, but this treatment decreases the depth of the excavation and flattens the chest.[33]

During treatment, a standard suction cup (3 sizes) or even a special shape for female patients with breasts is applied to the anterior chest wall that covers the pectus excavatum (**Fig. 7**). Vacuum is then applied to the cup, which elevates the chest wall. The cup should be used approximately 30 minutes twice a day during the beginning of treatment and can then be gradually increased to several hours every day. The length of the treatment varies but may extend up to several years. There are only a few clinical results published with this technique,[33,34] but the complication rate is low. Moderate pain often develops in the beginning of treatment and subcutaneous hematoma may develop that disappears after several hours.

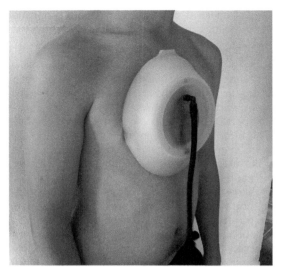

Fig. 7. A suction cup is applied to the anterior chest wall that covers the pectus excavatum for vacuum bell treatment.

Pectus-up

This is the newest minimal invasive technique, which has not yet been described in the literature, but has been presented at scientific meetings. Instead of the pectus excavatum being pushed from the inside by a pectus bar as in the Nuss procedure, the sternum is pulled to the correct position and fixed to an H-shaped metal plate with screws. The system is placed subcutaneously in front of the sternum. Consequently, surgical intervention in the mediastinum is avoided.

PECTUS CARINATUM
Introduction

In most areas of the world, pectus carinatum represents fewer than 10% of chest wall anomalies. In South America, however, it is claimed to be the most frequent chest wall deformity, although this has not been documented in the literature. Surgical correction was commonly performed by a modified open Ravitch technique until the minimal invasive procedure for pectus excavatum was published. Today, the treatment of pectus carinatum has also changed to a minimal noninvasive technique with a brace in most clinics that treat chest wall anomalies. The indication for correction is exclusively for cosmetic reasons, but some patients also complain of pain when they lie on their chest because of the prominent sternum.

Brace Treatment

As far back as 1979, Haje and Raymundo[35] published the first article on brace treatment of chest

wall anomalies, but it was published in a Brazilian medical journal and had little influence on clinical practice in the rest of the world. After Nuss introduced his minimally invasive technique for surgical repair of pectus excavatum, Abramson[36] from Argentina published a new technique whereby the carinatum was compressed by a subcutaneous bar. This technique caused more focus on the external compression, and today it is used in most departments that are interested in chest wall anomalies. The success of this technique rests on an inherent flexibility of the chest that allows adequate compression of the sternum over a period until it reaches a good position, similar to brace treatment of teeth. Complications are rare, but skin lesions were a problem previously. Since 2008, newer dynamic compression methods allow measurement of the pressure applied on the skin, which has reduced these lesions.[37]

Patient Selection

Clinical evaluation of the patient is all that is required before treatment. If the chest is too rigid, requiring more than 10 pounds per square inch (PSI) for compression, the brace technique is not possible and surgery is required either by the Abramson technique or by a modified Ravitch operation.

Technique

Both symmetric and asymmetric pectus carinatum may be corrected by this method. The patient is placed standing with the back against a wall and a pressure measurement tool is used on the sternum, which is compressed to its normal position (**Fig. 8**). The pressure needed for complete correction is recorded and named the "pressure for initial

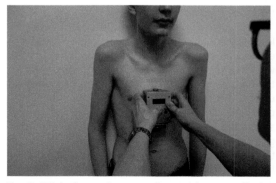

Fig. 8. With the patient standing against a wall. the sternum is compressed to its normal position and the pressure needed for complete correction is recorded (PIC).

correction" (PIC), which is measured in PSI units. Empirically, it was always suggested that the PIC should not exceed 10 PSI, even though anecdotal unpublished data suggest that a PIC as high as 14 PSI allows correction without complications. A custom-made brace (**Fig. 9**) is subsequently manufactured to fit the patient that allows constant pressure on the sternum. There are several different pads where the brace presses on the skin for different shapes of the anterior chest wall, so that the pressure from the brace may be delivered to a larger surface. When the brace has been adjusted to the patient, a "pressure of treatment" is set to approximately 3 PSI, which can be measured directly on the patient (**Fig. 10**). The patient is encouraged to wear the brace progressively as much as possible throughout the day and even during the night. The patient is seen in the outpatient clinic, every fourth week for adjustment of the "pressure of treatment," which gradually decreases when the sternum moves posteriorly from the treatment.

Depending on the PIC, the duration of treatment varies between 6 and 24 months. After complete correction, the patient should continue to wear the brace for approximately 6 months to retain the new position of the sternum. Many patients report moderate to severe pain when they begin the treatment, typically with a visual analog score (VAS) of up to 6 on a scale of 0 to 10 during the first days of treatment, but it gradually decreased to VAS 1 to 2 within the first week of treatment. Complications are few, but local hematomas or skin ulcerations may occur.

MINIMAL INVASIVE SURGICAL TREATMENT: THE ABRAMSON TECHNIQUE

In 2005, Abramson[36] published the first article about his technique of minimal invasive surgery for correction of pectus carinatum. Again, this

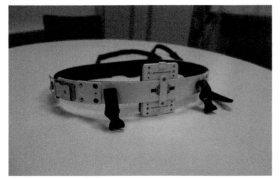

Fig. 9. A brace is fitted individually to each patient that allows constant pressure on the sternum.

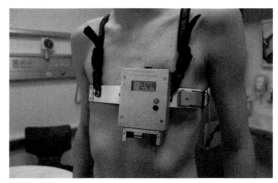

Fig. 10. When the brace has been adjusted to the patient, a "pressure of treatment" is set to approximately 3 PSI, which can be measured directly on the patient.

article was not published in English and did not have a widespread clinical implication in the English-speaking world, but an English article was published in 2009 with their experience in 40 patients.[38]

Patient Selection

This surgical method may be used in patients in whom the chest is too rigid to be corrected by the brace technique. It also may be used in patients with combined pectus excavatum and carinatum, similar to the unpublished sandwich technique described by Park.[39]

Preparation and Patient Positioning

The patient is placed supine with both arms abducted or flexed in front of the head. The procedure is performed under general anesthesia with single lumen intubation. Preoperative antibiotics are given and continued for 2 to 3 days depending on local tradition.

Surgical Approach

The most prominent point of the sternum is defined and a horizontal line through this is extended to both sides where 2 small transverse incisions are made in the midaxillary area. These are used for fixation plates to the ribs that will keep the compressor bar in position. Subperiosteal tunnels are dissected around 2 adjacent ribs for wire fixation of the plates. These plates should be strictly perpendicular to the horizontal line. The plates are only loosely fixed until the compressor bar has been attached. An extrathoracic tunnel is then dissected from one side to the other subcutaneously or beneath the pectoral muscle. The bar is bent according to the shape of the chest and guided through this tunnel by a rubber tube. When the bar is inserted in the plates, the sternum is compressed to the desired shape, the plates are fixed to the ribs, and the bar is fixed to the plates before the skin is closed.

Immediate Postoperative Care

The patient is extubated on the operating table and a postoperative chest radiograph is used to exclude perioperative pneumothorax, but if that occurs, most patients are treated conservatively without a chest tube unless the pneumothorax progresses or the patient develops shortness of breath, which is extremely rare.

Rehabilitation and Recovery

The postoperative pain is treated by epidural analgesia and per oral medication similar to the method described under pectus excavatum. The patients are mobilized immediately after surgery and typical length of stay in the hospital is 4 to 5 days.

Clinical Results

There are only a few published articles of this surgical technique,[38,40] but they report good cosmetic results with few complications. Complications have mainly been problems of the fixation to the ribs. Initial steel wires were used, but because of breakage, multifilament sutures are now used.

The bar is removed after 1 to 2 years.

Modifications

Modifications to the Abramson technique were published in 2009. Hock[41] used a complete "opposite" Nuss procedure that was performed without a thoracoscope. The bar ends were placed inside the chest cavity and the bar came in front of the sternum without a need for stabilizers. Hock's article[41] described only 5 patients, and it was necessary to reoperate 4 of them. Later the same year, Kálmán[42] published a modification in which the ends of the bar were placed outside the chest cavity, so the bar was lying under only 1 rib on each side. The operation was performed also without a thoracoscope. Results from 14 patients were good in all but 1 patient who needed a reoperation because of bar dislocation. In 2011, Perez and colleagues[43] published a modification but presented only 2 patients, in whom he used a combination of the techniques presented by Hock[41] and Kálmán[42] so that one end of the pectus bar was inside and the other end outside the chest.

REFERENCES

1. Brochhausen C, Turial S, Muller FK, et al. Pectus excavatum: history, hypotheses and treatment options. Interactive Cardiovasc Thorac Surg 2012;14(6):801–6.
2. Robicsek F, Watts LT. Surgical correction of pectus excavatum. How did we get here? Where are we going? Thorac Cardiovasc Surg 2011;59(1):5–14.
3. Ashrafian H. Leonardo da Vinci and the first portrayal of pectus excavatum. Thorax 2013;68(11):1081.
4. Bauhinus J. Observationum Medicariam. Liber II, Observ. Francfurti. 1600;Liber II, Observ. 264, Francfurti.
5. Meyer L. Zurchirurqishen Behandlung der augeborenen Trichterbrust. Verh Bel Med Gest 1911;42:364.
6. Ravitch MM. The operative treatment of pectus excavatum. Ann Surg 1949;129(4):429–44.
7. Nuss D, Kelly RE Jr, Croitoru DP, et al. A 10-year review of a minimally invasive technique for the correction of pectus excavatum. J Pediatr Surg 1998;33(4):545–52.
8. Chung CS, Myrianthopoulos NC. Factors affecting risks of congenital malformations. I. Analysis of epidemiologic factors in congenital malformations. Report from the Collaborative Perinatal Project. Birth Defects Orig Artic Ser 1975;11(10):1–22.
9. Redlinger RE Jr, Kelly RE, Nuss D, et al. Regional chest wall motion dysfunction in patients with pectus excavatum demonstrated via optoelectronic plethysmography. J Pediatr Surg 2011;46(6):1172–6.
10. Lesbo M, Tang M, Nielsen HH, et al. Compromised cardiac function in exercising teenagers with pectus excavatum. Interactive Cardiovasc Thorac Surg 2011;13(4):377–80.
11. Sacco Casamassima MG, Gause C, Goldstein SD, et al. Patient satisfaction after minimally invasive repair of pectus excavatum in adults: long-term results of Nuss procedure in adults. Ann Thorac Surg 2016;101(4):1338–45.
12. Kelly RE Jr, Cash TF, Shamberger RC, et al. Surgical repair of pectus excavatum markedly improves body image and perceived ability for physical activity: multicenter study. Pediatrics 2008;122(6):1218–22.
13. Krasopoulos G, Goldstraw P. Minimally invasive repair of pectus excavatum deformity. Eur J Cardiothorac Surg 2011;39(2):149–58.
14. Kelly RE Jr. Pectus excavatum: historical background, clinical picture, preoperative evaluation and criteria for operation. Semin Pediatr Surg 2008;17(3):181–93.
15. Jacobsen EB, Thastum M, Jeppesen JH, et al. Health-related quality of life in children and adolescents undergoing surgery for pectus excavatum. Eur J Pediatr Surg 2010;20(2):85–91.
16. Chao CJ, Jaroszewski DE, Kumar PN, et al. Surgical repair of pectus excavatum relieves right heart chamber compression and improves cardiac output in adult patients–an intraoperative transesophageal echocardiographic study. Am J Surg 2015;210(6):1118–24 [discussion: 1124–5].
17. Maagaard M, Tang M, Ringgaard S, et al. Normalized cardiopulmonary exercise function in patients with pectus excavatum three years after operation. Ann Thorac Surg 2013;96(1):272–8.

18. Nuss D. Recent experiences with minimally invasive pectus excavatum repair "Nuss procedure". Jpn J Thorac Cardiovasc Surg 2005;53(7):338–44.

19. Ewert F, Syed J, Kern S, et al. Symptoms in pectus deformities: a scoring system for subjective physical complaints. Thorac Cardiovasc Surg 2017; 65(1):43–9.

20. Park HJ, Sung SW, Park JK, et al. How early can we repair pectus excavatum: the earlier the better? Eur J Cardiothorac Surg 2012;42(4):667–72.

21. Kelly RE, Goretsky MJ, Obermeyer R, et al. Twenty-one years of experience with minimally invasive repair of pectus excavatum by the Nuss procedure in 1215 patients. Ann Surg 2010;252(6):1072–81.

22. Jaroszewski DE, Ewais MM, Chao CJ, et al. Success of minimally invasive pectus excavatum procedures (modified Nuss) in adult patients (≥30 years). Ann Thorac Surg 2016;102(3):993–1003.

23. Croitoru DP, Kelly RE Jr, Goretsky MJ, et al. Experience and modification update for the minimally invasive Nuss technique for pectus excavatum repair in 303 patients. J Pediatr Surg 2002;37(3):437–45.

24. Park HJ, Chung WJ, Lee IS, et al. Mechanism of bar displacement and corresponding bar fixation techniques in minimally invasive repair of pectus excavatum. J Pediatr Surg 2008;43(1):74–8.

25. Tedde ML, de Campos JR, Wihlm JM, et al. The Nuss procedure made safer: an effective and simple sternal elevation manoeuvre. Eur J Cardiothorac Surg 2012;42(5):890–1.

26. Haecker FM, Sesia SB. Intraoperative use of the vacuum bell for elevating the sternum during the Nuss procedure. J Laparoendosc Adv Surg Tech A 2012;22(9):934–6.

27. Pilegaard HK. Nuss technique in pectus excavatum: a mono-institutional experience. J Thorac Dis 2015; 7(Suppl 2):S172–6.

28. Park HJ, Kim KS, Lee S, et al. A next-generation pectus excavatum repair technique: new devices make a difference. Ann Thorac Surg 2015;99(2):455–61.

29. Park HJ, Jeong JY, Kim KT, et al. Hinge reinforcement plate for adult pectus excavatum repair: a novel tool for the prevention of intercostal muscle strip. Interactive Cardiovasc Thorac Surg 2011;12(5):687–91.

30. Knudsen MR, Nyboe C, Hjortdal VE, et al. Routine postoperative chest X-ray is unnecessary following the Nuss procedure for pectus excavatum. Interactive Cardiovasc Thorac Surg 2013;16(6):830–3.

31. Neviere R, Montaigne D, Benhamed L, et al. Cardiopulmonary response following surgical repair of pectus excavatum in adult patients. Eur J Cardiothorac Surg 2011;40(2):e77–82.

32. Schaarschmidt K, Lempe M, Schlesinger F, et al. Lessons learned from lethal cardiac injury by Nuss repair of pectus excavatum in a 16-year-old. Ann Thorac Surg 2013;95(5):1793–5.

33. Haecker FM. The vacuum bell for conservative treatment of pectus excavatum: the Basle experience. Pediatr Surg Int 2011;27(6):623–7.

34. Lopez M, Patoir A, Costes F, et al. Preliminary study of efficacy of cup suction in the correction of typical pectus excavatum. J Pediatr Surg 2016;51(1):183–7.

35. Haje SA, Raymundo JLP. Considerações sobre deformidades da parede torácica anterior e apresentação de tratamento conservador para as formas com componentes de protrusão. Rev Bras Ortop 1979; 14(4):167–78.

36. Abramson H. A minimally invasive technique to repair pectus carinatum. Preliminary report. Arch Bronconeumol 2005;41(6):349–51 [in Spanish].

37. Martinez-Ferro M, Fraire C, Bernard S. Dynamic compression system for the correction of pectus carinatum. Semin Pediatr Surg 2008;17(3):194–200.

38. Abramson H, D'Agostino J, Wuscovi S. A 5-year experience with a minimally invasive technique for pectus carinatum repair. J Pediatr Surg 2009;44(1): 118–23 [discussion: 123–4].

39. Park HJ, Kim KS. The sandwich technique for repair of pectus carinatum and excavatum/carinatum complex. Ann Cardiothorac Surg 2016;5(5):434–9.

40. Yuksel M, Bostanci K, Evman S. Minimally invasive repair of pectus carinatum using a newly designed bar and stabilizer: a single-institution experience. Eur J Cardiothorac Surg 2011;40(2):339–42.

41. Hock A. Minimal access treatment of pectus carinatum: a preliminary report. Pediatr Surg Int 2009; 25(4):337–42.

42. Kalman A. Initial results with minimally invasive repair of pectus carinatum. J Thorac Cardiovasc Surg 2009;138(2):434–8.

43. Perez D, Cano JR, Quevedo S, et al. New minimally invasive technique for correction of pectus carinatum. Eur J Cardiothorac Surg 2011;39(2):271–3.

Straight Back Syndrome

Cameron D. Wright, MD

KEYWORDS

- Straight back syndrome • Tracheal obstruction • Chest wall deformity

KEY POINTS

- Straight back syndrome may rarely cause tracheal obstruction.
- Operative repair requires removal or thinning of the manubrium to relieve tracheal compression.
- Rarely the brachiocephalic artery also may be a cause of tracheal compression and require rerouting.

Straight back syndrome (SBS) is a rare congenital chest wall deformity such that the normal dorsal curvature of the thoracic spine is absent and instead is straight. This anatomic variant then effectively narrows the space between the posterior aspect of the manubrium and the anterior thoracic spine. This condition is often accompanied by pectus excavatum. If the loss of thoracic inlet space is severe enough, tracheal compression may ensue and lead to dyspnea. An additional cause of tracheal compression can be the brachiocephalic artery as it crosses the trachea in a narrowed space. Most patients with SBS do not have tracheal compression and do not exhibit respiratory symptoms but with extreme anterior spine displacement airway obstruction can occur.

SBS is most commonly associated with cardiac abnormalities, such as mitral valve prolapse and "pseudo-heart disease."[1,2] Patients can present with atypical chest pain, dyspnea, and palpitations. Approximately two-thirds of patients are found to have mitral valve prolapse either clinically or by echocardiography. One report described a patient with exertional pulmonary hypertension due to elevated pulmonary venous pressure due to compression of the left atrium and pulmonary veins from the narrow anterior-posterior chest.[3]

SBS causing airway compression severe enough to require operative treatment is so rare that in general there are only occasional case reports. We reported 4 patients in conjunction with our French colleagues several years ago.[4] In a general way, there are several possibilities to enlarge the space behind the upper sternum, including removing or thinning the manubrium, distracting the manubrium, elevating a severe pectus excavatum, or performing osteotomies of the anterior upper thoracic spine.

Each case is unique and an operative plan must necessarily be individualized. The computed tomography (CT) scan is the most important diagnostic modality and must be studied to identify points of airway compression and for possibilities for treatment. Our general philosophy was that it is less morbid to move the sternum than to remove the anterior portions of the offending vertebral bodies. Operations may be staged to gauge the results of an operative intervention if the initial procedure is thought likely to correct most of the airway compression. If the brachiocephalic artery is going to be divided and moved, it is prudent to study the circle of Willis to ensure that it is intact to minimize the risk of a watershed ischemic event.

Although each case is unique, a typical a classic case is illustrated in **Figs. 1–5**. The patent was a 21-year-old man with a long history of wheezing and dyspnea thought to be due to asthma. He had a mild pectus excavatum. His forced expiratory volume in 1 second was reduced at 37% of predicted. He eventually had a diagnosis of SBS.

Disclosures: None.
Division of Thoracic Surgery, Massachusetts General Hospital, Harvard Medical School, 55 Fruit Street, Boston, MA, 02114, USA
E-mail address: cdwright@partners.org

Thorac Surg Clin 27 (2017) 133–137
http://dx.doi.org/10.1016/j.thorsurg.2017.01.006
1547-4127/17/© 2017 Elsevier Inc. All rights reserved.

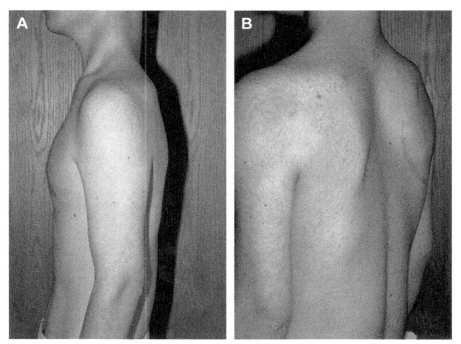

Fig. 1. A patient with SBS. Notice the narrow chest and the straight thoracic spine. (*A*) Lateral view (*B*). Posterior view. (*From* Grillo HC, Wright CD, Dartvelle PG, et al. Tracheal compression caused by straight back syndrome, chest wall deformity and anterior spine displacement: techniques for relief. Ann Thorac Surg 2005;80:2058; with permission.)

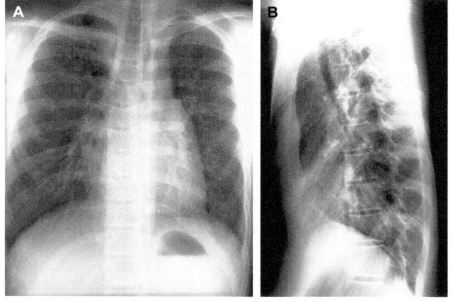

Fig. 2. A patient with SBS who required operation for tracheal compression (same as **Fig. 1**). (*A*) Chest radiograph anterior-posterior view demonstrating clear lung fields and slightly widened trachea. (*B*) Lateral view demonstrates a narrow chest with no dorsal curvature of the thoracic spine. (*From* Grillo HC, Wright CD, Dartvelle PG, et al. Tracheal compression caused by straight back syndrome, chest wall deformity and anterior spine displacement: techniques for relief. Ann Thorac Surg 2005;80:2059; with permission.)

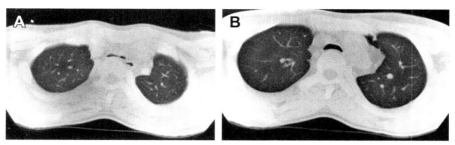

Fig. 3. CT scan of the patient from **Fig. 1** at the thoracic inlet. The trachea is severely compressed between the manubrium and the spine. (*A*) Axial image from upper thoracic inlet. (*B*) Axial image from just below thoracic inlet. (*From* Grillo HC, Wright CD, Dartvelle PG, et al. Tracheal compression caused by straight back syndrome, chest wall deformity and anterior spine displacement: techniques for relief. Ann Thorac Surg 2005;80:2060; with permission.)

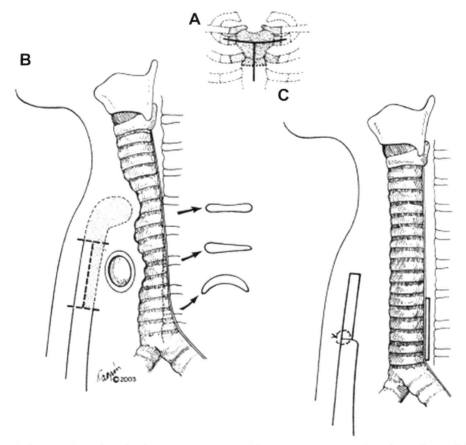

Fig. 4. Surgical correction of tracheal compression caused by severe SBS in patient from **Fig. 1**. (*A*) Incision centered over the manubrium. (*B*) Lateral diagram demonstrating the points of compression. The tracheal lumen is illustrated at each point of compression. The upper trachea is pinched between the manubrium and the spine. The brachiocephalic artery compresses the trachea lower down. The lower trachea is splayed and compressed against the spine. (*C*) Operative correction. The obstructing manubrium and brachiocephalic artery have been removed. The artery was transplanted laterally and the lower trachea was splinted with polypropylene mesh. The manubrium was thinned and used as a bone graft to protect the upper chest. (*D*) The brachiocephalic artery was transplanted with a graft to the right of the trachea. (*From* Grillo HC, Wright CD, Dartvelle PG, et al. Tracheal compression caused by straight back syndrome, chest wall deformity and anterior spine displacement: techniques for relief. Ann Thorac Surg 2005;80:2060; with permission.)

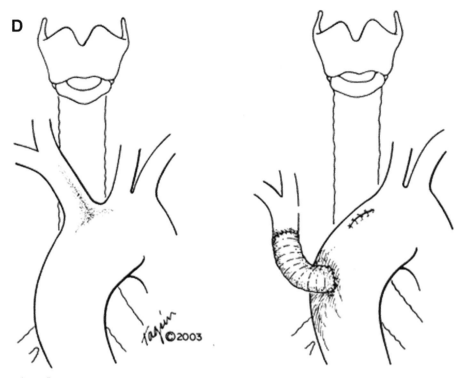

Fig. 4. (*continued*)

He slowly declined over 3 years and developed worsening stridor, ultimately to the severity he required intubation. He was transferred to our hospital intubated. His physique is illustrated in **Fig. 1**. His chest radiograph is shown in **Fig. 2** and demonstrates his narrow chest and straight thoracic vertebral column. The chest CT is shown in **Fig. 3** and shows severe anterior-posterior compression of the trachea from forward displacement of the vertebral column. The operation required to improve the patient is illustrated in **Fig. 4**. Briefly, the manubrium was removed to relieve the compression of the trachea and the brachiocephalic artery was rerouted so that it was not compressing the trachea. The removed manurial plate was thinned and wired back in place to protect the upper chest contents but fashioned such that it did not compress the trachea. Depending on the anatomy and patient, other options exist, including not replacing the manubrium at all (similar to a mediastinal tracheostomy), using a sandwich of methyl-methacrylate and polypropylene mesh, polytetrafluoroethylene, or a metal strut. Rarely, malacic tracheal segments require

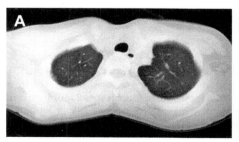
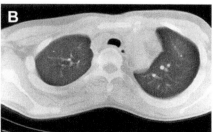

Fig. 5. CT scan of patient from **Figs. 1–3** after operative correction. Note the improvement in size of the tracheal lumen. (*A*) Axial image from upper thoracic inlet. (*B*) Axial image from just below thoracic inlet. (*From* Grillo HC, Wright CD, Dartvelle PG, et al. Tracheal compression caused by straight back syndrome, chest wall deformity and anterior spine displacement: techniques for relief. Ann Thorac Surg 2005;80:2061; with permission.)

resection at a later date if identified as causing obstruction. Results cannot be generalized, as these cases are so rare, but if a thoughtful operative plan is carried out to relieve tracheal compression, good results are expected.

REFERENCES

1. Davies MK, Mackintosh P, Cayton RM, et al. The straight back syndrome. Q J Med 1980;49:443–60.
2. Ansari A. The straight back syndrome. Clin Cardiol 1985;8:290–305.
3. Leinbach RC, Hawthorne JW, Dinsmore RE. Straight back syndrome with pulmonary venous obstruction. Am J Cardiol 1968;21:588–92.
4. Grillo HC, Wright CD, Dartvelle PG, et al. Tracheal compression caused by straight back syndrome, chest wall deformity and anterior spine displacement: techniques for relief. Ann Thorac Surg 2005; 80:2057–62.

Management of Primary Soft Tissue Tumors of the Chest Wall

Anthony Cipriano, MD, William Burfeind Jr, MD*

KEYWORDS

- Surgery • Chest wall tumors • Malignancy

KEY POINTS

- Primary chest wall tumors compose only 1% to 2% of all thoracic neoplasms and approximately 60% are malignant. A majority of patients present with a painless mass.
- Work-up includes thoracic imaging with CT, MRI, and possibly PET. Diagnosis is made with a carefully designed core needle biopsy or incisional biopsy.
- Surgical wide excision with negative margins is the standard treatment of most primary soft tissue malignancies.

INTRODUCTION

The chest wall comprises a variety of tissues, including skin, fat, lymphovascular vessels, fascia, muscle, bone, and cartilage. Overall, it provides protection to vital organs, provides stability for the shoulders and arms during movement, and has evolved into a dynamic structure that assists with respiration. Chest wall masses have broad potential etiologies and present diagnostic and therapeutic challenges. Each of the tissue types composing the chest wall can give rise to benign or malignant primary chest wall masses. Also, due to the chest wall's close proximity to the breast, pleura, mediastinum, and lung, it is at risk from invasion from locally advanced tumors and inflammatory processes. Finally, the chest wall is a large target for metastases from distant tumors and these are the most common malignant chest wall masses.

Primary chest wall tumors compose only 1% to 2% of all thoracic neoplasms.[1] They are best classified according to their tissue of origin (bone or soft tissue) and are further subdivided as either benign or bearing malignant potential. Approximately 60% of primary chest wall tumors are malignant, with increasing malignant risk at the extremes of age.[2] Of these malignant tumors, approximately 55% arise from bone or cartilage and 45% from soft tissue.[3] All chest wall tumors are uncommon and their nomenclature varies throughout the literature. This article reviews the most common primary soft tissue chest wall tumors and focuses on their description, demographics, diagnosis, treatment, and general prognosis.

DIAGNOSIS

A majority of patients with a primary soft tissue chest wall tumor present with a painless, palpable mass. Often, patients have already undergone some form of thoracic imaging for unrelated conditions and a chest wall mass was noticed incidentally. Rapid growth and pain are harbingers of malignant tumor behavior and imply local invasion of adjacent structures, such as periosteal or neurologic structures. There are no reliable clinical

Disclosure Statement: The authors have nothing to disclose.
Department of Surgery, St. Luke's University Health Network, Bethlehem, PA 18015, USA
* Corresponding author. 701 Ostrum Street, Suite 603, Bethlehem, PA 18015.
E-mail address: William.Burfeind@sluhn.org

features, however, for distinguishing benign from malignant. Initial work-up should include obtaining a detailed history with attention to prior/current malignancies, radiation exposure, recent/current infections, symptoms associated with the mass (ie, pain), time of discovery, rate of growth, and review of prior thoracic imaging. If the mass is palpable, its size and characteristics of soft versus hard and fixed versus mobile should be noted. The initial goal of evaluation and work-up of a chest wall mass should be to determine if it is a primary or secondary lesion because this guides treatment.

Diagnostic imaging cannot reliably distinguish benign from malignant lesions although it can be suggestive of tumor type and differentiating benign from malignant tumors. The advent of cross-sectional imaging techniques, such as CT and MRI, have aided in localizing and determining the extent of chest wall lesions. Chest radiography is often the initial test and does not allow for comprehensive tumor assessment. CT is more sensitive than chest radiography for detecting calcified tumor matrix and cortical destruction—findings suggestive of extracompartmental extension—and delineating the extent of pleural, lung, mediastinal, and nodal involvement.[4] MRI is useful for further characterization of the lesion and offers superior spatial resolution giving precise delineation of tissue planes including bone and vasculature. The imaging features of many chest wall tumors can be suggestive but often are nonspecific.

PET has proved a valuable tool in the evaluation, particularly in regard to staging and response to treatment, of various neoplasms and has shown promise in the imaging of chest wall tumors as well. With regard to sarcomas, PET has been shown more accurate than CT alone in initial staging, evaluation of early treatment response, and both short-term and long-term follow-up.[5] Furthermore, when combined with CT, accuracy in staging, treatment response evaluation, and restaging is increased compared with either PET or CT alone.[5] For restaging sarcomas, PET has been shown to detect high-grade local recurrence, with a sensitivity of 88% and specificity of 92%.[6] It also has a role in distinguishing high-grade soft tissue sarcomas from low-grade sarcomas/benign lesions (95% sensitivity and 75% specificity).[7] PET has found superior to CT for defining the extent of chest wall sarcomas, particularly for tumors greater than 5.5 cm, and may provide some value in planning full-thickness chest wall resection.[8] In 1 study of pediatric patients, ages 18 or less, PET and conventional imaging modalities (CIMs) have been shown equally effective in

detection of primary tumors (accuracy 100%).[9] In the same study, PET was superior to CIMs for the detection of lymph node involvement (sensitivity 95% vs 25%, respectively) and bone manifestations (sensitivity 90% vs 57%, respectively). Best results were obtained with combined modalities, with 91% correct therapeutic decisions, a rate significantly better than using CIMs alone (59%). The role of PET/CT in regard to evaluating chest wall tumors is promising, but the evidence is not strong enough to support its use as a sole modality for pretherapeutic staging. It adds useful information, however, when combined with CT and MRI.

Whether a tissue diagnosis is needed prior to definitive therapy depends mainly on the size of the lesion. Small lesions (<2 cm), thought to be benign, should undergo excisional biopsy with clear, greater than 1 cm, margins, which is both diagnostic and therapeutic. If the lesion is larger (>2 cm) or likely malignant, a preoperative tissue diagnosis is preferred. Fine-needle aspirate is acceptable when a metastatic lesion is suspected but often yields insufficient tissue to adequately diagnose and grade soft tissue sarcomas.[1,10,11] If a lesion is benign, it is resected with negative margins and, if malignant, wide excision is performed.[12] It is essential to plan biopsies with future curative resection in mind because re-excision of the biopsy tract is required as part of the definitive resection.

Benign Soft Tissue Tumors

Lipoma

Lipomas are benign mesenchymal tumors of adipose tissue that can occur superficially and deep as well as intramuscularly.[13] They are painless, nontender, well-circumscribed, mobile masses that can occur extra thoracically or intrathoracically.[14] Intrathoracic lipomas can remain completely intrathoracic or can extend through the ribs, giving rise to a dumbbell-shaped lesion.[15,16] The appearance of these tumors on CT and MRI shows a well-circumscribed, homogeneous lesion with the imaging characteristics of fat, which distinguishes it from liposarcomas that almost always contain inhomogeneous nonfatty elements.[17] Grossly, these lesions are well-circumscribed, thinly encapsulated tumors of mature adipose tissue. Histologically, they comprise uniform, mature adipose tissue that lacks atypia or multivaculolated lipoblasts.[13] Malignant transformation is exceedingly rare.[18] Surgical excision is indicated for cosmetic purposes or if malignancy cannot be excluded (**Table 1**).[1]

Table 1
Primary benign chest wall soft tissue neoplasms by tissue of origin

Vascular	Hemangioma
	Glomus tumor
	Lymphangioma
Peripheral nerve	Schwannoma
	Neurofibroma
	Ganglioneuroma
	Paraganglioma
Adipose	Lipoma
	Spindle cell lipoma
Fibrous/histiocytic	Desmoid
	Granuloma
Muscular	Rhabdomyoma

Lipoblastoma

Lipoblastoma is a benign mesenchymal tumor of the embryonic white fat tissue with 80% to 90% seen in patients less than 3 years of age.[19–21] They are nonmetastasizing lesions that have a 14% rate of local recurrence and tend to mature with the patient rather than undergo malignant transformation[22]; 80% of lipoblastomas occur in the extremities, and involvement of the chest wall, pleura, and parenchyma is limited to a few dozen case reports.[23,24] Treatment is by wide resection.[25]

Hemangioma

Soft tissue hemangiomas are benign vascular neoplasms that can arise in the subcutaneous, intermuscular, intramuscular, or synovial tissues and are usually detected by the third decade of life.[26,27] Clinical manifestations include a palpable mass, subtle bulging, pain, or a combination of these signs and symptoms.[27] Soft tissue hemangiomas are uncommon in the chest wall.[28] CT scan demonstrates a poorly defined mass with attenuation approximating that of skeletal muscle, along with phleboliths and underlying bone remodeling.[17] The lesion characteristically demonstrates intermediate signal intensity on T1-weighted MRI and marked hyperintensity on T2-weighted images.[17] The standard treatment of deep soft tissue hemangiomas is complete surgical excision. Radiotherapy, cryotherapy, embolization, electrocoagulation, and injection of sclerosing agents may be beneficial in cases of unresectable or partially resected lesions.[29] Local recurrence occurs in up to 18% of patients after resection.[30]

Benign peripheral nerve sheath tumors: neurofibromas/schwannomas

Benign peripheral nerve sheath tumors consist of schwannomas and neurofibromas and originate from the myelin nerve sheath or nerves, respectively. One retrospective review of 60 patients with neurogenic tumors of the chest found 63% of the neurogenic tumors originated in the mediastinum and 27% in the chest wall, with schwannomas the most common type (85%).[31] Schwannomas are encapsulated neoplasms that typically occur in patients between 20 years and 50 years of age. On contrast CT, they appear as homogenous masses and can reveal multiple patterns, such as multiple cystic and hypodense areas, radial enhancement, peripheral enhancement with low attenuated center, diffuse low attenuation, or central enhancement with peripheral hypodensity.[32] The signal intensity of schwannoma on T1-weighted MRI is equal to or slightly greater than that of muscle and on T2 is markedly greater.[33] Neurofibromas are the most common benign tumors to arise from peripheral nerves and may occur alone or in association with neurofibromatosis 1 (NF1).[34] They often occur between 20 years and 30 years of age and are slow growing, may or may not have a capsule, and can include components of cystic degeneration and calcification.[33] A characteristic imaging feature of neurofibroma on MRI is the target sign (hyperintense rim with centrally decreased intensity on T2-weighted images), which, if present, can help differentiate neurofibromas from malignant peripheral nerve sheath tumors.[35,36] Neurofibromas associated with NF1 undergo malignant transformation in 10% to 20% of cases.[11,17] Apart from NF1, the frequency of neurogenic tumors harboring malignancy is low and is reported to be from 4% to 13%.[37] Imaging is often helpful in the diagnosis of benign peripheral nerve sheath tumors, and resection is usually reserved for symptomatic or rapidly enlarging lesions.

Desmoid tumors

Of the benign soft tissue chest wall tumors, desmoid tumors, also termed fibromas, deserve special attention. They are considered a type of low-grade malignant sarcoma due to their tendency to invade local structures and their high rate of local recurrence. Despite the local aggressiveness of desmoid tumors, they do not metastasize. They are derived from fibroblasts in fascia, muscle aponeurosis, or muscle striae (**Fig. 1**A). These tumors can be seen in association with familial syndromes, such as familial adenomatous polyposis, and in scars caused from trauma or prior surgical incisions. Chest wall desmoids account for 8% to 10% of all desmoid tumors and frequently present as a slowly enlarging mass in the anterior chest wall or shoulder girdle.[38,39]

The CT findings of desmoid tumors are variable and depend on the collagen content and the

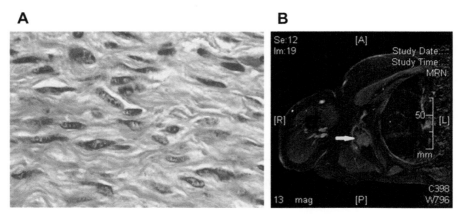

Fig. 1. (A) Streaming bundles of elongated spindle cells set in a stroma of pink collagen. The tumor cells contain uniform bland nuclei. The absence of cytologic atypia and varied rates of mitosis are classic features of desmoid tumors. (Hematoxylin and eosin, original magnification ×400). (B) MRI demonstrating a solid, enhancing tumor in the right axilla/chest wall (*arrow*), measuring 1.5 cm × 2.1 cm × 2.3 cm. This is located anterior to the inferior tip of the scapular wing, within the substance of the subscapularis muscle.

amount of solid or necrotic tissue present. Higher solid tissue content correlates with greater enhancement on CT scan.[4] Desmoids have similar intensity to muscle on T1 and central areas of low signal surrounded by very high signal on T2-weighted MRI[4] (**Fig. 1**B). Most lesions are confined by the surrounding fascia and can displace or surround adjacent structures.[40]

The principles of biopsy remain the same, with the recommendation that larger tumors undergo incisional biopsy with careful attention paid to incision orientation.[39] The gold standard treatment of patients with desmoid tumor is excision to negative margins; however, the margin width has not been standardized. For chest wall desmoids, resection of a normal rib above and below the tumor with 5-cm clear margins has been advocated.[39] Margin status has been an inconsistent predictor of recurrence. One study from 2004 demonstrated that the local recurrence rate is 89% with positive surgical margins and less than 20% with negative margins,[41] whereas other studies have failed to demonstrate a relationship between margin positivity and recurrence.[42] Recurrence is most common within 12 months after resection and unlikely if patients are disease-free after 5 years.[43] Radiotherapy is used as an adjunct to surgery in cases of R2 resection or, primarily, if excision would cause unacceptable morbidity. Sherman and colleagues[44] reported on the results of a 20-year follow-up after using radiotherapy for treatment of desmoid tumors in 45 patients: 14 had inoperable lesions or gross residual disease after resection, and 31 patients received postoperative radiation for positive margins. After 20 years, tumor-free status was present

in 71% of patients treated with radiation alone and 77% of patients receiving radiation in conjunction with resection. More recently, observation has become an option for some desmoids. This recommendation is based on the results of a retrospective analysis that found that small, asymptomatic desmoids could be safely observed, especially if they were located in sites where an increase in growth would not impact resectability.[45]

Malignant Soft Tissue Tumors

Sarcomas

Most malignant soft tissue tumors of the chest wall are sarcomas, **Table 2**, and a few select histologic types are highlighted later. They can be classified into 7 diagnostic categories: muscular, vascular, fibrous, peripheral nerve, adipose, hematologic, and cutaneous. There are approximately 13,000 new cases of soft tissue sarcomas diagnosed annually in the United States and less than 10% arise in the chest wall.[46,47] Most present as a painless chest wall mass with a mean duration of 12 months.[48] With treatment by resection alone, overall 5-year survival is approximately 66%, with 5-year survival for high-grade tumors significantly less than those with low-grade histology, 49% versus 90%, respectively.[49] Metastases develop in 10% of patients with low-grade tumors and 50% in those with high-grade tumors.[11] Prognostic factors for patients with primary soft tissue sarcomas of the chest wall are inconsistent in literature series; however, adequate surgical resection is still considered the most important factor in achieving a survival advantage. The other consistent independent prognostic factor along with the

Table 2
Primary malignant chest wall soft tissue neoplasms by tissue of origin

Muscular	Leiomyosarcoma
	Rhabdomyosarcoma
Vascular	Angiosarcoma
Fibrous/histiocytic	Malignant fibrous histiocytoma
	Aggressive fibromatosis
Peripheral nerve	Neuroblastoma
	Ganglioneuroblastoma
	Neurofibrosarcoma/ malignant peripheral Nerve sheath tumors
Adipose	Liposarcoma
Hematologic	Malignant lymphoma
	Extraosseous solitary myeloma
Cutaneous	Dermatofibrosarcoma protuberans
Other	SS

type of surgical resection performed is histologic tumor grade with high-grade tumor status conferring a worse prognosis.[48,49]

Malignant fibrous histiocytoma

Malignant fibrous histiocytoma (also known as malignant fibrous xanthoma, fibroxanthosarcoma, and undifferentiated pleomorphic sarcoma) develops in the deep soft tissues of the extremities, trunk, retroperitoneum, or chest wall and is the most common soft tissue sarcoma in adults.[48] Most occur between ages 50 and 70 years.[50] When seen in the chest wall, it is often in the setting of prior radiation exposure.[51] In an analysis of 200 patients with malignant fibrous histiocytoma, 2-year survival was 60%, recurrence rate 44%, and metastatic rate 42%, and prognosis was related to depth and size of the initial tumor.[52] Older reviews report a 5-year survival of only 38%.[53] On CT scan, it manifests as a nonspecific heterogeneously enhancing mass in muscle and fascial planes with ill-defined contours.[4] Diagnosis is typically made with an incisional biopsy and treatment is with wide excision. Stages II and III disease may involve preoperative or postoperative radiation therapy or chemotherapy.[54]

Synovial sarcoma

The designation of synovial sarcoma (SS) is a misnomer because these tumors have no relation to synovium but do often present as a heterogeneous soft tissue mass in close proximity to joints. They have been reported to occur in the thorax but

are extremely rare in the chest wall.[55] They most commonly occur between the ages of 20 years and 40 years and present as a deep-seated, slow-growing mass with or without pain. Grossly, SS infiltrates irregularly into adjacent soft tissue, does not have a capsule, and can have peripheral satellite nodules (**Fig. 2**A).[56] A helpful diagnostic feature of SS is the presence of calcification that is noted radiographically in as many as 30% of tumors.[57] The most common radiographic finding, however, of SS involving the chest wall is a heterogeneously enhancing soft tissue mass with well-defined margins without calcification (**Fig. 2**B).[58] Prognosis is reportedly poor, with 5-year survival approaching 50%, and factors that predict a worse prognosis are tumor size greater than 5 cm, male gender, age greater than 20, extensive tumor necrosis/hemorrhage, high grade, greater than 10 mitotic figures per 10 high-power fields, and neurovascular invasion.[59] Local control is achieved with adequate excision to negative margins, adjuvant radiation, adjuvant chemotherapy, and metastasectomy.[54] SS has been found sensitive to ifosfamide and doxorubicin, with 24% response rates.[60]

Rhabdomyosarcoma

Rhabdomyosarcoma arises from primitive mesenchymal cells committed to become striated muscle and is the most common pediatric soft tissue sarcoma; however, it is rare in the chest wall.[61] Most cases are stage III or stage IV at presentation, with only 10% completely resectable[62,63]; 40% of patients present with metastasis so a complete staging work-up should be done before considering primary resection.[62] Preoperative work-up should include an MRI of the primary tumor as well as bone scans and PET/CT to rule out metastatic disease.[25] In the largest published retrospective series for chest wall rhabdomyosarcoma, Hayes-Jordan and colleagues[62] reviewed data from 130 patients enrolled in the Intergroup Rhabdomyosarcoma Study protocols, versions I through IV. All 130 patients reviewed had the chest wall as the primary tumor site. Median follow-up was 12.1 years, median age was 9 years (0–20 years), 37% of patients had alveolar histology, and 39% of patients presented with stage IV disease. All patients who presented without metastasis had a 5-year overall survival of 61% compared with 7% for metastatic patients (P<.001). They found no significant difference in 5-year overall survival in patients who had a complete resection, complete resection with positive microscopic margins, or biopsy/partial resection only, with 5-year survival rates of 65%, 60%, and 59% respectively. This review showed that

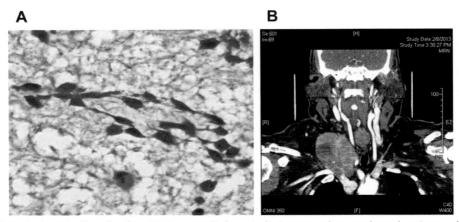

Fig. 2. (*A*) Fascicular spindle cells of an SS. Tumor cells have indistinct cytoplasm and overlapping nuclei and are associated with wiry collagenous stroma. (Hematoxylin and eosin, original magnification ×400). (*B*) Coronal CT image of an 8.8 cm × 4.1 cm × 5.8 cm SS. This heterogeneous soft tissue mass centered within the right supraclavicular region extends into the right lung apex and anterior cervical triangle.

complete surgical resection before or after induction chemotherapy does not significantly change 5-year survival and that there is no survival advantage to chest wall tumor excision with positive compared with negative margins. Treatment algorithms vary by institution and are in constant flux; however, traditional management is first an assessment of initial resectability. If the mass appears resectable with a high likelihood of achieving negative margins, resection is performed. If removal of the mass would cause untoward morbidity or if a microscopic negative margin is unlikely, incisional biopsy is done, followed by induction chemotherapy and radiotherapy, followed by restaging, and followed by surgical resection and then adjuvant chemotherapy and radiotherapy as indicated.[64] Patients with alveolar histology benefit from radiotherapy irrespective of postsurgical status.[65]

Fibrosarcoma

Fibrosarcoma develops from the connective tissue found in structures of the thorax and usually occurs in the chest wall and lungs of adults.[66] They are seen as heterogeneous in attenuation and signal intensity on CT and MRI, respectively, due to internal necrosis and hemorrhage.[67] Treatment of chest wall fibrosarcoma is wide excision.

PRINCIPLES OF SURGERY

The foundation of treatment of most primary chest wall tumors is surgical resection. Resection must ensure negative margins because a positive margin is the most important risk factor for local recurrence and can potentially have an impact on survival.[68] When positive surgical margins are

encountered, reresection should be highly considered if it will not lead to undue functional impairment.[69] Required margin length is controversial. A 4-cm margin recommendation for malignant chest wall tumors came from a 1986 report of 90 patients undergoing chest wall resection for primary chest wall tumors, where patients with resection margins of 2 cm had a 5-year disease free survival of 29% compared with patients with 4-cm resection margins, 56%.[53] This did not reach significance ($P<.06$), however. Current consensus guidelines suggest that a margin of at least 1 cm is adequate although closer margins may be necessary to preserve major neurovascular structures.[54] Lymph node dissection should only be performed in the presence of obvious disease.[70] Benign lesions should be resected to microscopically clear margins. Proper oncologic resection should not be compromised by concern over tumor size or site because myocutaneous flaps and prosthetic materials make chest wall reconstruction feasible in most instances.

CHEMOTHERAPY AND RADIATION THERAPY FOR SARCOMAS

Surgery alone is the standard treatment of superficial, low-grade tumors that are less than 5 cm and amenable to resection with adequate margins. This approach can achieve over a 90% local control rate.[71] Some patients, however, are at high risk of recurrence, both locally and systemically, and may benefit from adjunctive treatments.[72] Common adverse factors that predict recurrence include histology, tumor grade, tumor size, deep location, positive resection margin, and patient age.[73] Patients with high-risk tumors should be evaluated in a multidisciplinary setting and be enrolled in clinical trials, if possible.

Radiation therapy for nonextremity sarcomas is used to reduce the incidence of local recurrence. Radiation therapy can be given either preoperatively or postoperatively with equal efficacy. Preoperative therapy, however, is associated with higher rates of wound complications, whereas postoperative radiation therapy is associated with worse long-term functional outcomes.[74] Postoperative radiation therapy is also recommended if resection margins are positive. Postoperative radiation therapy decreases local recurrence rates in patients with marginal resections or positive margins.[75] Recent practice guidelines recommend considering radiation therapy, either preoperatively or postoperatively (category I recommendation), in stage II and stage III extremity and trunk sarcomas.[54]

Numerous trials have been completed to evaluate the effects of chemotherapy in soft tissue sarcomas. In the only randomized trial to compare preoperative chemotherapy with surgery alone in high-risk tumors, there was no difference in either disease-free survival or overall survival.[76] At least 20 clinical trials and 3 pooled analyses have examined adjuvant chemotherapy in soft tissue sarcomas and results are mixed. In 2008, a meta-analysis of 1953 patients with soft tissue sarcomas demonstrated an overall survival benefit to adjuvant chemotherapy (hazard ratio 0.77; 95% CI, 0.64–0.93; $P = .01$).[77] In a pooled analysis of 2 large European phase III trials (N = 819), however, doxorubicin-based adjuvant chemotherapy was not associated with an overall survival advantage except in patients with R1 resections.[78] Current treatment guidelines reflect the uncertainty about adjuvant chemotherapy and give it a category 2B recommendation in stage II and stage III extremity and trunk soft tissue sarcomas.[54]

SUMMARY

Primary chest wall tumors are rare and represent a challenging clinical entity for surgeons and oncologists. Preoperative work-up includes a thorough history, radiographic imaging, and a thoughtful biopsy approach that will not make a future definitive resection more difficult. Treatment decisions are based predominantly on tumor histology, stage, local aggressiveness, and responsiveness to chemotherapy and radiation. Wide excision is the foundation of treatment of most malignant primary chest wall tumors. The role of radiation therapy in the neoadjuvant or adjuvant setting is to reduce local recurrence. The use of adjuvant chemotherapy is more controversial. For most primary chest wall malignancies, margin-negative resection remains the best chance of cure.

REFERENCES

1. Faber LP, Somers J, Templeton AC. Chest wall tumors. Curr Probl Surg 1995;32(8):661–747.
2. Pass HI. Primary and metastatic chest wall tumors. In: Roth JA, Ruckdeschel JC, Weisenburger TH, editors. Thoracic oncology. 2nd edition. Philadelphia: W.B. Saunders; 1995. p. 519–37.
3. Burt M. Primary malignant tumors of the chest wall. The Memorial Sloan-Kettering Caner Center experience. Chest Surg Clin N Am 1994;4:137–54.
4. Tateishi U, Gladish GW, Kusumoto M, et al. Chest wall tumors: radiologic findings and pathologic correlation. Part 2: malignant tumors. Radiographics 2003;23:1491–508.
5. Piperkova E, Mikhaeil M, Mousavi A, et al. Impact of PET and CT in PET/CT studies for staging and evaluating treatment response in bone and soft tissue sarcomas. Clin Nucl Med 2009;34(3):146–50.
6. Schwarzbach M, Dimitrakopoulou-Strauss A, Willeke F, et al. Clinical value of [18-F] flurodeoxyglucose positron emission tomography imaging in soft tissue sarcomas. Ann Surg 2000;231(3):380–6.
7. Lucas JD, O'Doherty MJ, Cronin BF, et al. Prospective evaluation of soft tissue masses and sarcomas using Flurodeoxyglucose positron emission tomography. Br J Surg 1999;86:550–6.
8. Petermann D, Allenbach G, Schmidt S, et al. Value of positron emission tomography in full-thickness chest wall resections for malignancies. Interact Cardiovasc Thorac Surg 2009;9:406–10.
9. Volker T, Denecke T, Steffen I, et al. Positron emission tomography for staging of pediatric sarcoma patients: results of a prospective multicenter trial. J Clin Oncol 2007;25(34):5435–41.
10. Sabanathan S, Shah R, Mearns AJ. Surgical treatment of primary malignant chest wall tumors. Eur J Cardiothorac Surg 1999;11:1011–6.
11. Anderson BO, Burt ME. Chest wall neoplasms and their management. Ann Thorac Surg 1994;58: 1774–81.
12. Kucharczuk JC. Chest Wall Mass. ACS Surgery: principles and practice 2005; 1–6.
13. Bassett MD, Schuetze SM, Disteche C, et al. Deep-seated, well differentiated lipomatous tumors of the chest wall and extremities. Cancer 2005;103(2): 409–16.
14. Sulzer MA, Goei R, Bollen EC, et al. Lipoma of the external thoracic wall. Eur Respir J 1994;7:207–9.
15. Faer MJ, Burnam RE, Beck CL. Transmural thoracic lipoma: demonstration by computed tomography. AJR Am J Roentgenol 1978;130:161–3.
16. Heuer GJ. The thoracic lipomas. Ann Surg 1933;98: 801–19.

17. Jeung M, Gangi A, Gasser B, et al. Imaging of Chest wall disorders. Radiographics 1999;19:617–37.

18. Enzinger EM, Weiss SW. Soft tissue tumors. 2nd edition. St Louis (MO): Mosby Co; 1988. p. 3–328.

19. Mognato G, Cecchetto G, Carli M, et al. Is surgical treatment of lipoblastoma always necessary? J Pediatr Surg 2000;35:1511–3.

20. Chung EB, Enzinger FM. Benign lipoblastomatosis: an analysis of 35 cases. Cancer 1973;32:482–91.

21. Coffin CM. Lipoblastoma: an embryonal tumor of soft tissue related to organogenesis. Semin Diagn Pathol 1994;11:98–103.

22. Coffin CM, Dehner LP. Soft tissue tumours in the first year of life: a report of 190 cases. Pediatr Pathol 1990;10:509–26.

23. Kanu A, Oermann CM, Malicki D, et al. Pulmonary lipoblastoma in an 18 month old child: a unique tumor in children. Pediatr Pulmonol 2002;34:150–4.

24. Samuel M, Moore E, Burge DM. Thoracic wall lipoblastoma: a case report and review of histopathology and cytogenetics. Eur J Pediatr Surg 2000;10: 53–7.

25. Watt AJB. Chest wall lesions. Pediatr Respir Rev 2002;3(4):328–38.

26. DeFilippo JL, Yu JS, Weis L, et al. Soft tissue hemangioma with adjacent periosteal reaction simulating a primary bone tumor. Skeletal Radiol 1996; 167:683–7.

27. Ly JQ, Sanders TG. Case 65: Hemangioma of the Chest wall. Radiology 2003;229:726–9.

28. Yonehara Y, Nakatsuka T, Ichioka I, et al. Intramuscular haemangioma of the anterior chest wall. Br J Plast Surg 2000;53:257–9.

29. Griffo S, Stassano P, De Luca G, et al. Intramusular hemangioma of the chest wall: an unusual tumor. J Thorac Cardiovasc Surg 2007;134:1368–9.

30. Cohen AJ, Youkey JR, Claggett GP, et al. Intramuscular hemangioma. JAMA 1983;249:2680–2.

31. Yamaguchi M, Yoshino I, Fukuyama S, et al. Surgical treatment of neurogenic tumors of the chest. Ann Thorac Cardiovasc Surg 2004;10(3):148–51.

32. Ko SF, Lee TY, Lin JW, et al. Thoracic neurilemmomas: an analysis of computed tomography findings in 36 patients. J Thorac Imaging 1998;13:21–6.

33. Tateishi U, Gladish GW, Kusumoto M, et al. Chest wall tumors: RAdiolgic findings and pathological correlation: part 1 Benign tumors. Radiographics 2003;23:1477–90.

34. Kransforf MJ. Benign soft-tissue tumors in a large referral population: distribution of specific diagnoses by age, sex, and location. AJR Am J Roentgenol 1995;164:395–402.

35. Kuhlman JE, Bouchardy L, Fishman EK, et al. CT and MR imaging evaluation of chest wall disorders. Radiographics 1994;14:571–95.

36. Bhargava R, Parham DM, Lasater OE, et al. MR imaging differentiation of benign and malignant peripheral nerve sheath tumors: use of the target sign. Pediatr Radiol 1997;27:124–9.

37. Reeder LB. Neurogenic tumors of the mediastinum. Semin Thorac Cardiovasc Surg 2000;12:261–7.

38. Brodsky JT, Gordon MS, Hajdu SI, et al. Desmoid tumors of the chest wall. A locally recurrent problem. J Thorac Cardiovasc Surg 1992;104(4):900–3.

39. Allen PJ, Shriver CD. Desmond tumors of the chest wall. Semin Thorac Cardiovasc Surg 1999;11(3):264–9.

40. O'Sullivan P, O'Dwyer H, Flint J, et al. Soft tissue tumours and mass-like lesions of the chest wall: a pictorial review of CT and MR findings. Br J Radiol 2007;80:574–80.

41. Abbas AE, Deschamps C, Cassivi SD, et al. Chest wall desmoid tumors: results of surgical intervention. Ann Thorac Surg 2004;78:1219.

42. Gronchi A, Casali PG, Mariani L, et al. Quality of surgery and outcomes in extra-abdominal aggressive fibromatosis: a series of patients surgically treated at a single institution. J Clin Oncol 2003;21:1390–7.

43. Posner M, Shiu MH, Newsome JL, et al. The desmoid tumor: not a benign disease. Arch Surg 1989;124:191–6.

44. Sherman NE, Romsdahl M, Evans H, et al. Desmoid tumor: a 20 year radiotherapy experience. Int J Radiat Oncol Biol Phys 1990;19:37–40.

45. Bonvalot S, Eldweny H, Haddad V, et al. Extra-abdominal primary fibromatosis: aggressive management could be avoided in a subgroup of patients. Eur J Surg Oncol 2008;34:462–8.

46. Toro JR, Travis LB, Wu HJ, et al. Incidence patterns of soft tissue sarcomas, regardless of primary site, in the surveillance, epidemiology and end results program, 1978-2001: an analysis of 26,758 cases. Int J Cancer 2006;119(12):2922–30.

47. Brennan MF, Alektiar KM, Maki RG. Soft tissue sarcoma. In: De Vita JR, Hellman S, Rosenberg AS, editors. Cancer: principles & practice of oncology. 6th edition. Philadelphia: Lippincot-Raven Publishers; 2001. p. 1841–90.

48. Gross JL, Younes RN, Haddad FJ, et al. Soft-tissue sarcomas of the chest wall: prognostic factors. Chest 2005;127:902–8.

49. Gordon MS, Hajdu SI, Bains MS, et al. Soft tissue sarcomas of the chest wall. Results of surgical resection. J Thorac Cardiovasc Surg 1991;101(5): 843–54.

50. Gallo AE, Coady MA. Chest wall tumors. In: Yuh DD, Vricella LA, Baumgartner WA, editors. The Johns Hopkins manual of cardiothoracic surgery. New York: McGraw-Hill Professional; 2006. p. 80.

51. Souba WW, McKenna RJ Jr, Meis J, et al. Radiation-induced sarcomas of the chest wall. Cancer 1986; 57:610–5.

52. Weiss SW, Enzinger FM. Malignant fibrous histiocytoma: an analysis of 200 cases. Cancer 1978;41: 2250–66.

53. King RM, Pairolero PC, Trastek VF, et al. Primary chest wall tumors: factors affecting survival. Ann Thorac Surg 1986;41:597–601.

54. National Comprehensive Cancer Network. Soft tissue sarcomas (version 2.2016). Available at: https://www.nccn.org/professionals/physician_gls/pdf/sarcoma.pdf. Accessed July 30, 2016.

55. Nicholson AG, Goldstraw P, Fisher C, et al. Synovial sarcoma of the pleura and its differentiation from other primary pleural tumors: a clinicopathologic and immunohistochemical review of three cases. Histopathology 1998;33:508–13.

56. Fisher C. Synovial Sarcoma. Ann Diagn Pathol 1998; 2(6):401–21.

57. Siegel MJ. Magnetic resonance imaging of musculo-skeletal soft tissue masses. Radiol Clin North Am 2001;39:701–20.

58. Duran-Menducti A, Costello P, Vargas SO. Primary synovial sarcoma of the chest: radiographic and clinicopathologic correlation. J Thorac Imaging 2003;18:87–93.

59. Dennison S, Weppler E, Giacoppe G, et al. Primary pulmonary synovial sarcoma: a case report and review of current diagnostic and therapeutic standards. Oncologist 2004;9:339–42.

60. Spillane AJ, A'Hern R, Judson IR, et al. Synovial Sarcoma: a clinicopathologic, staging, and prognostic assessment. J Clin Oncol 2000;18:3794–803.

61. Berg H, Rijn RR, Merks J. Management of tumors of the chest wall in childhood: a review. J Pediatr Hematol Oncol 2008;30(3):214–21.

62. Hayes-Jordan A, Stoner JA, Anderson JR, et al. The impact of surgical excision in chest wall rhabdomyo-sarcoma: a report from the children's oncology group. J Pediatr Surg 2008;43:831–6.

63. Andrassy RJ, Wiener ES, Raney RB, et al. Thoracic sarcomas in children. Ann Surg 1998;227:170–3.

64. Saenz NC, Ghavimi F, Gerald W, et al. Chest wall rhabdomyosarcoma. Cancer 1997;80:1513–7.

65. Wolden SL, Anderson JR, Crist WM, et al. Indications for radiotherapy and chemotherapy after complete resection in rhabdomyosarcoma: a report from the Intergroup Rhabdomyosarcoma Sutdies I to III. J Clin Oncol 1999;17:3468–75.

66. Cakir O, Topal U, Bayram AS, et al. Sarcomas: rare primary malignant tumors of the thorax. Diagn Interv Radiol 2005;11:23–7.

67. Gladish GW, Sabloff BM, Munden RF, et al. Primary thoracic sarcomas. Radiographics 2002;22:621–37.

68. Perry RR, Venzon D, Roth JA, et al. Survival after surgical resection for high-grade chest wall sarcomas. Ann Thorac Surg 1990;49:363.

69. Zagars GK, Ballo MT, Pisters PW, et al. Surgical margins and reresection in the management of patients with soft tissue sarcoma using conservative surgery and radiation therapy. Cancer 2003;97: 2544–53.

70. Fong Y, Coit DG, Woodruff JM, et al. Lymph node metastasis from soft tissue sacoma in adults. Analysis of data from a prospective database of 1772 sarcoma patients. Ann Surg 1993;217(1):72.

71. Pisters PW, Pollock RE, Lewis VO, et al. Long-term results of a prospective trial of surgery alone with selective use of radiation for patients with T1 extremity and trunk soft tissue sarcomas. Ann Surg 2007; 246(4):675.

72. Cahlon O, Brennan MF, Jia X, et al. A prospective nomogram for local recurrence risk in extremity soft tissue sarcomas after limb-sparing surgery without adjuvant radiation. Ann Surg 2012; 255(2):343.

73. Trovik CS, Bauer HC, Alvegrad TA, et al. Surgical margins, local recurrence and metastasis in soft tissue sarcomas: 559 surgically treated patients from the Scandinavian Sarcoma Group Register. Eur J Cancer 2000;36(6):710–6.

74. Zagars GK, Ballo MT, Pisters WT, et al. Preoperative vs. postoperative radiation therapy for soft tissue sarcoma: a retrospective comparative evaluation of disease outcome. Int J Radiat Oncol Biol Phys 2003;56:482–8.

75. Khanfir K, Alzieu L, Terrier P, et al. Does adjuvnt radiatin therapy increase loco-regional control after optimal resection of soft-tissue sarcoma of the extremity. Eur J Cancer 2003;39(13):1872–80.

76. Gortzak E, Azzarelli A, Buesa J, et al. A randomised phase II study on neo-adjuvant chemotherapy for 'high-risk' adult soft-tissue sarcoma. Eur J Cancer 2001;37:1096–103.

77. Pervaiz N, Colterjohn N, Farrokhyar F, et al. A systematic meta- analysis of randomized controlled trials of adjuvant chemotherapy for localized resectable soft-tissue sarcoma. Cancer 2008; 113:573–81.

78. Le Cesne A, Ouali M, Leahy MG, et al. Doxorubicin-based adjuvant chemotherapy in soft tissue sarcoma: pooled analysis of two STBSG- EORTC phase III clinical trials. Ann Oncol 2014;25:2425–32.

Management of Lung Cancer Invading the Superior Sulcus

Johannes R. Kratz, MD[a],*, Gavitt Woodard, MD[b],
David M. Jablons, MD[c]

KEYWORDS

- Superior sulcus • Pancoast • Non–small cell lung cancer • Apical • Tumor

KEY POINTS

- The first cases series of superior sulcus tumors was reported by Dr Pancoast, a radiologist, in the early twentieth century.
- For decades, superior sulcus tumors were thought to be distinct category of slow-growing lung cancers. They are now recognized, however, as non–small cell lung cancers that are distinct from nonapical tumors in their location only and not their biology.
- Modern treatment is centered around neoadjuvant chemoradiotherapy followed by surgical resection with the goal of achieving complete pathologic response and R0 resection.

HISTORY

There is an unusual but apparently infrequent type of intrathoracic growth occurring in the apical region, yet found with sufficient frequency in my experience to warrant a collective report of the cases encountered.
—Henry K. Pancoast, MD[1]

In 1924, Dr Pancoast described a series of patients with apical intrathoracic tumors in his landmark case series.[1] A radiologist by training, Dr Pancoast documented 5 instances of apical shadows on chest radiograph (CXR) that were diagnosed as intrathoracic tumors, either pathologically or clinically.[1] Despite the pathologic diagnosis of lung cancer in 1 of these tumors, Dr Pancoast concluded that these apical tumors were either pleural endotheliomas or sarcomas in origin.[1]

Dr Pancoast went on to become the first president of the American Board of Radiology.[2] In 1932, he gave a chairman's address at the annual session of the American Medical Association.[3] In his address, he described 7 total cases of "superior sulcus pulmonary tumors."[3] These superior sulcus tumors shared the following key characteristics: (1) an apical shadow along with posterior destruction of 1 or more of the first 3 ribs on CXR and (2) a distinct clinical presentation now commonly referred to as Pancoast syndrome.[3] This syndrome was described in his address as shoulder and arm pain in the C8-T2 distribution, wasting of the hand muscles, and Horner syndrome on the affected side.[3]

Unbeknownst to Dr Pancoast, one of his contemporaries, Dr Tobias, described the same clinical lesion and symptoms in 1932.[4] Unlike Dr Pancoast, Dr Tobias correctly identified the origin

---

Disclosure: The authors have no relevant commercial or financial interests to disclose.
[a] Department of Thoracic Surgery, University of California, San Francisco, Box 0118, San Francisco, CA 94143-0118, USA; [b] Department of Surgery, University of California, San Francisco, Box 0470, 513 Parnassus Avenue, 321, San Francisco, CA 94122, USA; [c] Department of Thoracic Surgery, University of California, San Francisco, 1600 Divisadero Street, Room A-743, San Francisco, CA 94143-1724, USA
* Corresponding author.
E-mail address: johannes.kratz@ucsf.edu

of these tumors as bronchogenic carcinomas.[4,5] In subsequent decades, the origin of these superior sulcus tumors was confirmed by other investigators as primary lung cancer.[6–10]

DEFINITION

All patients in Dr Pancoast's original case series presented with Pancoast syndrome.[1,3] Subsequent investigators also only included patients with superior sulcus tumors associated with classic symptoms in their case series reports.[10–13] As treatment paradigms began to change and surgical resection became an important component of multimodality therapy, investigators began to include any patients with apical lung cancers in their studies regardless of Pancoast syndrome, leading to inconsistent use of the term, *superior sulcus tumor*.[14–21] The lack of consistency led Detterbeck[8] to propose a formal definition of superior sulcus tumors in 2003. Detterbeck defined a superior sulcus tumor as a "lung cancer arising in the apex of the lung that involves structures of the apical chest wall," regardless of symptoms.[8] In his proposal, the apical chest wall was defined as the level of the first rib or higher. Chest wall structures included the parietal pleura, ribs, vertebral bodies, vessels, nerves, and nerve roots.[8] The American College of Chest Physicians has subsequently endorsed this definition as have other modern investigators.[5–7,22] The term, superior sulcus tumor, was rejected by many investigators in the decades that followed Dr Pancoast's landmark articles because the superior sulcus was not considered an embryologic or anatomic structure.[23] In modern literature, however, the terms, *Pancoast tumor*, *Pancoast-Tobias tumor*, and *superior sulcus tumor*, are now used interchangeably.[5–9,22]

CLINICAL PRESENTATION

It has been estimated that superior sulcus tumors represent less than 5% of patients with lung cancer.[22] One prospective database study identified superior sulcus tumors in 3.2% of patients with newly diagnosed lung cancer.[15] The incidence of lung cancer in the United States has been estimated at 228,190 cases per year.[24] Based on these numbers, it can be estimated that approximately 7300 patients present with superior sulcus tumors per year in the United States.

Almost all patients who present with a superior sulcus tumor are symptomatic. In 2 reported series that detailed the presenting symptoms of patients, the numbers of asymptomatic patients were only 5% and 1.5%, respectively.[14,15] The most common reported symptom is shoulder pain.[9,10,14,15,25] One

study that looked at 139 patients who underwent surgical resection over 16 years at a single institution reported that 127 (91.4%) of patients presented with shoulder pain.[14] In another study, 107 of 131 patients (82%) with superior sulcus tumors presented with shoulder pain. As originally described by Dr Pancoast, shoulder pain commonly radiates to the arm, axilla, or scapula.[14] Different compartments may give rise to different presentations of arm pain. Pain in the anterior chest wall, shoulder and upper limb, and axillary distributions are typical of anterior, middle, and posterior compartment tumors, respectively.[26] Approximately 25% of patients present with Horner syndrome (24%–32% in the case series discussed previously[14]). Only approximately 10% of patients present with classic Pancoast syndrome (shoulder/arm pain, Horner syndrome, and hand muscle wasting).[10] Other less common symptoms include hemoptysis, weight loss, pneumonia, dysphonia, superior vena cava syndrome, and paraneoplastic syndromes.[5,9,10,14,15]

DIAGNOSIS

In his original case series, Dr Pancoast described the difficulty of identifying superior sulcus tumors on plain CXR, noting that a majority of tumors in his series were missed on initial interpretation of the CXR.[1] Although CXR remains important in incidental detection of or initial screening for superior sulcus tumors, any clinical suspicion for a superior sulcus tumor should be investigated with higher-resolution imaging studies. A reasonable first test to establish a diagnosis of superior sulcus tumor is a high-resolution, contrast-enhanced chest CT scan.[27] Chest CT not only can establish a diagnosis of superior sulcus tumor but also provide information on regional lymph node and thoracic metastases.[27] In addition, despite the multitude of imaging options available today, contrast-enhanced CT remains the best modality to assess tumor involvement of 2 specific structures. First, it provides superior visualization of bony invasion involving the ribs and thoracic spine.[27,28] Second, contrast-enhanced CT provides excellent resolution of the upper thoracic vascular structures that may be invaded by tumor.[27]

In the past several decades, the use of MRI in assessing superior sulcus tumors has become widespread.[27–29] MRI provides superior assessment of tumor extension into the surrounding soft tissues.[27–29] In particular, MRI is the best modality to detect tumor involvement with the brachial plexus nervous system as well as the vertebral foramina and spinal cord.[27] For this reason, it is currently the imaging modality of

first rib is mobilized by dividing the first rib costo-chondral cartilage.[56]

An alternative anterior approach involves a hemiclamshell thoracotomy with or without suprasternal (trapdoor) extension[5,49,51] (**Fig. 3**). The incision starts vertically in the sternal midline and is extended laterally in the third or fourth interspace toward the axilla in an L-shaped fashion.[49,51] Anterior approaches to superior sulcus tumors that involve the vertebrae may necessitate a second posterior incision,[5] often as a staged procedure.[49] Excellent descriptions of various anterior approaches have been published by Macchiarini,[57] de Perrot,[54] and Dartevelle and Mentzer.[51]

Minimally invasive approaches to resection of the superior sulcus tumor are currently being developed.[58–60] Cheung and Lim[59] reported on their experience with a video-assisted thoracic surgery (VATS)-assisted resection of a 7-cm tumor located in the posterior thoracic inlet. After a standard VATS right upper lobectomy, this group completed the chest wall resection by performing a small posterolateral-paravertebral thoracotomy.[59] A limited anterior, clavicle-sparing approach followed by VATS lobectomy has also been described.[60] Finally, several robotic-assisted resections of superior sulcus tumors have been performed by Cerfolio at the University

of Alabama, Birmingham (personal communication, 2016). It is reasonable to expect that the number of minimally invasive superior sulcus tumor resections will grow as more and more groups attempt to expand the indications and use of minimally invasive VATS and robotic thoracic surgery.

SUMMARY

Superior sulcus tumors have posed a formidable therapeutic challenge since their original description by Pancoast and Tobias in the early twentieth century. Today, the standard of care is trimodality therapy consisting of induction chemoradiotherapy followed by surgery with the dual goals of complete pathologic response and R0 resection. The evolution of treatment approaches over time has provided outcomes that come increasingly closer to rivaling those of similarly staged nonapical lung cancer.[37] Further advances in improving both the morbidity and mortality associated with superior sulcus tumors will likely come in the form of improved medical therapy, such as targeted therapy or immunotherapy, as well as minimally invasive approaches to surgical resection. More research is needed in both areas to keep advancing knowledge and treatment of superior sulcus tumors.

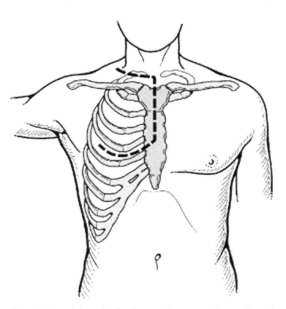

Fig. 3. Hemiclamshell thoracotomy with optional suprasternal (trapdoor) extension. The incision starts vertically in the sternal midline and is extended laterally in the third or fourth interspace toward the axilla in an L-shaped fashion. (*From* Macchiarini P. Resection of superior sulcus carcinomas (anterior approach). Thorac Surg Clin 2004;14(2):229–40; with permission.)

REFERENCES

1. Pancoast HK. Importance of careful roentgen-ray investigations of apical chest tumors. J Am Med Assoc 1924;83:1407–11.
2. Olson JS. The history of cancer: an annotated bibliography. New York: Greenwood Press; 1989.
3. Pancoast HK. Superior pulmonary sulcus tumor: tumor characterized by pain, horner's syndrome, destruction of bone and atrophy of hand muscles. J Am Med Assoc 1932;99:1391–6.
4. Tobias JW. Sindrome ápico-costo-vertebral doloroso por tumor apexiano: su valor diagnóstico en el cáncer primitivo pulmonar. Rev Med Lat Am 1932;19:1552–6.
5. Rusch VW. Management of pancoast tumours. Lancet Oncol 2006;7:997–1005.
6. Kozower BD, Larner JM, Detterbeck FC, et al. Special treatment issues in non-small cell lung cancer. Chest 2013;143:e369S–99S.
7. Glassman LR, Hyman K. Pancoast tumor: a modern perspective on an old problem. Curr Opin Pulm Med 2013;19:340–3.
8. Detterbeck FC. Changes in the treatment of Pancoast tumors. Ann Thorac Surg 2003;75:1990–7.
9. Arcasoy SM, Jett JR. Superior pulmonary sulcus tumors and Pancoast's syndrome. N Engl J Med 1997;337:1370–6.

10. Hilaris BS, Luomanen RK, Beattie EJ. Integrated irradiation and surgery in the treatment of apical lung cancer. Cancer 1971;27:1369–73.

11. Paulson DL. The importance of defining location and staging of superior pulmonary sulcus tumors. Ann Thorac Surg 1973;15:549–51.

12. Hilaris BS, Luomanen RK, Mahan GD, et al. Interstitial irradiation of apical lung cancer. Radiology 1971; 99:655–60.

13. Shaw RR, Paulson DL, Kee JL. Treatment of superior sulcus tumor by irradiation followed by resection. Ann Surg 1961;154:29–40.

14. Martinod E, D'Audiffret A, Thomas P, et al. Management of superior sulcus tumors: experience with 139 cases treated by surgical resection. Ann Thorac Surg 2002;73:1534–9 [discussion: 1539–40].

15. Millar J, Ball D, Worotniuk V, et al. Radiation treatment of superior sulcus lung carcinoma. Australas Radiol 1996;40:55–60.

16. Okubo K, Wada H, Fukuse T, et al. Treatment of Pancoast tumors. Thorac Cardiovasc Surg 1995;43: 284–6.

17. Fuller DB, Chambers JS. Superior sulcus tumors: combined modality. Ann Thorac Surg 1994;57: 1133–9.

18. Ginsberg RJ, Martini N, Zaman M, et al. Influence of surgical resection and brachytherapy in the management of superior sulcus tumor. Ann Thorac Surg 1994;57:1440–5.

19. Sartori F, Rea F, Calabrò F, et al. Carcinoma of the superior pulmonary sulcus. Results of irradiation and radical resection. J Thorac Cardiovasc Surg 1992;104:679–83.

20. Neal CR, Amdur RJ, Mendenhall WM, et al. Pancoast tumor: radiation therapy alone versus preoperative radiation therapy and surgery. Int J Radiat Oncol Biol Phys 1991;21:651–60.

21. Wright CD, Moncure AC, Shepard JA, et al. Superior sulcus lung tumors. Results of combined treatment (irradiation and radical resection). J Thorac Cardiovasc Surg 1987;94:69–74.

22. Peedell C, Dunning J, Bapusamy A. Is there a standard of care for the radical management of non-small cell lung cancer involving the apical chest wall (Pancoast tumours)? Clin Oncol (R Coll Radiol) 2010;22:334–46.

23. Teixeira JP. Concerning the Pancoast tumor: what is the superior pulmonary sulcus? Ann Thorac Surg 1983;35:577–8.

24. Siegel R, Naishadham D, Jemal A. Cancer statistics, 2013. CA Cancer J Clin 2013;63:11–30.

25. Marulli G, Battistella L, Mammana M, et al. Superior sulcus tumors (Pancoast tumors). Ann Transl Med 2016;4:239.

26. Panagopoulos N, Leivaditis V, Koletsis E, et al. Pancoast tumors: characteristics and preoperative assessment. J Thorac Dis 2014;6(Suppl 1):S108–15.

27. Bruzzi JF, Komaki R, Walsh GL, et al. Imaging of non-small cell lung cancer of the superior sulcus: part 2: initial staging and assessment of resectability and therapeutic response. Radiographics 2008;28: 561–72.

28. Takasugi JE, Rapoport S, Shaw C. Superior sulcus tumors: the role of imaging. J Thorac Imaging 1989;4:41–8.

29. Beale R, Slater R, Hennington M, et al. Pancoast tumor: use of MRI for tumor staging. South Med J 1992;85:1260–3.

30. Iezzi A, Magarelli N, Carriero A, et al. Staging of pulmonary apex tumors. Computerized tomography versus magnetic resonance. Radiol Med 1993;88: 24–30 [in Italian].

31. Heelan RT, Demas BE, Caravelli JF, et al. Superior sulcus tumors: CT and MR imaging. Radiology 1989;170:637–41.

32. Rapoport S, Blair DN, McCarthy SM, et al. Brachial plexus: correlation of MR imaging with CT and pathologic findings. Radiology 1988;167:161–5.

33. Collaud S, Waddell TK, Yasufuku K, et al. Long-term outcome after en bloc resection of non-small-cell lung cancer invading the pulmonary sulcus and spine. J Thorac Oncol 2013;8:1538–44.

34. Kernstine KH, Moon J, Kraut MJ, et al. Trimodality therapy for superior sulcus non-small cell lung cancer: Southwest Oncology Group-Intergroup Trial S0220. Ann Thorac Surg 2014;98:402–10.

35. Gomez DR, Cox JD, Roth JA, et al. A prospective phase 2 study of surgery followed by chemotherapy and radiation for superior sulcus tumors. Cancer 2012;118:444–51.

36. Cruz CSD, Tanoue LT, Matthay RA. Lung cancer: epidemiology, etiology, and prevention. Clin Chest Med 2011;32:605–44.

37. Detterbeck FC, Boffa DJ, Tanoue LT. The new lung cancer staging system. Chest 2009;136:260–71.

38. Marulli G, Battistella L, Perissinotto E, et al. Results of surgical resection after induction chemoradiation for Pancoast tumours. Interact Cardiovasc Thorac Surg 2015;20:805–11 [discussion: 811–2].

39. Li J, Dai C-H, Shi S-B, et al. Induction concurrent chemoradiotherapy compared with induction radiotherapy for superior sulcus non-small cell lung cancer: a retrospective study. Asia Pac J Clin Oncol 2010;6:57–65.

40. Kunitoh H, Kato H, Tsuboi M, et al. Phase II trial of preoperative chemoradiotherapy followed by surgical resection in patients with superior sulcus non-small-cell lung cancers: report of Japan Clinical Oncology Group trial 9806. J Clin Oncol 2008;26: 644–9.

41. Walker JE. Superior sulcus pulmonary tumor (Pancoast syndrome). J Med Assoc Ga 1946;35:364.

42. Chardack WM, Maccallum JD. Pancoast syndrome due to bronchiogenic carcinoma: successful

surgical removal and postoperative irradiation; a case report. J Thorac Surg 1953;25:402–12.

43. Chardack WM, Maccallum JD. Pancoast tumor; five-year survival without recurrence or metastases following radical resection and postoperative irradiation. J Thorac Surg 1956;31:535–42.

44. Ginsberg RJ, Rubinstein LV. Randomized trial of lobectomy versus limited resection for T1 N0 non-small cell lung cancer. Lung Cancer Study Group. Ann Thorac Surg 1995;60:615–22 [discussion: 622–3].

45. Rusch VW, Giroux DJ, Kraut MJ, et al. Induction chemoradiation and surgical resection for non-small cell lung carcinomas of the superior sulcus: Initial results of Southwest Oncology Group Trial 9416 (Intergroup Trial 0160). J Thorac Cardiovasc Surg 2001;121: 472–83.

46. Wright CD, Menard MT, Wain JC, et al. Induction chemoradiation compared with induction radiation for lung cancer involving the superior sulcus. Ann Thorac Surg 2002;73:1541–4.

47. Rusch VW, Giroux DJ, Kraut MJ, et al. Induction chemoradiation and surgical resection for superior sulcus non-small-cell lung carcinomas: long-term results of Southwest Oncology Group Trial 9416 (Intergroup Trial 0160). J Clin Oncol 2007;25:313–8.

48. Marra A, Eberhardt W, Pöttgen C, et al. Induction chemotherapy, concurrent chemoradiation and surgery for Pancoast tumour. Eur Respir J 2007;29: 117–26.

49. Donington J, Vaillères E, Bains M, et al. Management of the apical tumor: May 4, 2013, Minneapolis, MN. Semin Thorac Cardiovasc Surg 2013;25: 256–71.

50. Niwa H, Masaoka A, Yamakawa Y, et al. Surgical therapy for apical invasive lung cancer: different approaches according to tumor location. Lung Cancer 1993;10:63–71.

51. Dartevelle P, Mentzer SJ. Anterior approach to superior sulcus tumors. Oper Tech Thorac Cardiovasc Surg 2006;11:154–63.

52. Kent MS, Bilsky MH, Rusch VW. Resection of superior sulcus tumors (posterior approach). Thorac Surg Clin 2004;14:217–28.

53. Cuadrado DG, Grogan EL. Management of superior sulcus tumors: posterior approach. Oper Tech Thorac Cardiovasc Surg 2011;16:154–66.

54. de Perrot M. Resection of superior sulcus tumors: anterior approach. Oper Tech Thorac Cardiovasc Surg 2011;16:138–53.

55. Dartevelle PG, Chapelier AR, Macchiarini P, et al. Anterior transcervical-thoracic approach for radical resection of lung tumors invading the thoracic inlet. J Thorac Cardiovasc Surg 1993;105:1025–34.

56. Grunenwald D, Spaggiari L. Transmanubrial osteomuscular sparing approach for apical chest tumors. Ann Thorac Surg 1997;63:563–6.

57. Macchiarini P. Resection of superior sulcus carcinomas (anterior approach). Thorac Surg Clin 2004; 14:229–40.

58. Caronia FP, Fiorelli A, Ruffini E, et al. A comparative analysis of Pancoast tumour resection performed via video-assisted thoracic surgery versus standard open approaches. Interact Cardiovasc Thorac Surg 2014;19:426–35.

59. Cheung IH, Lim E. Video-assisted thoracoscopic surgical lobectomy with limited en bloc resection of superior sulcus tumor. J Thorac Cardiovasc Surg 2012;144:e148–51.

60. Linden PA. Video-assisted anterior approach to Pancoast tumors. J Thorac Cardiovasc Surg 2010;140: e38–9.

Management of Breast Cancer Invading Chest Wall

Boris Sepesi, MD, FACS

KEYWORDS

- Breast cancer • Chest wall • Resection • Reconstruction • Surgical management

KEY POINTS

- Surgical treatment of locally advanced or recurrent breast cancer involving the chest wall continues to play a role in the therapeutic armamentarium as part of the multidisciplinary treatment regimen.
- Significant progress has been made in chest wall reconstructive techniques.
- Advancements in understanding cancer biology and behavior, and the development of novel therapeutic agents expanded therapeutic options.
- Patient selection and superb knowledge of the most recent and effective treatment regimens are necessary to maximize the survival benefit and quality of life for patients affected with breast cancer involving the chest wall.

INTRODUCTION

Breast cancer affects 1 in 8 women (∼12% lifetime risk), and it is the second leading cause of cancer-related death (21.5 deaths per 100,000) among women, following lung cancer.[1] In 2016, an estimated 246,660 new cases of invasive breast cancer are expected to be diagnosed in the United States, not including 61,000 new carcinoma in situ diagnoses.[1] Fortunately, the death rates from breast cancer have been decreasing since early 1990s mainly due to increased awareness, earlier detection, and treatment advancements. Depending on the stage of the disease at the time of diagnosis, current therapeutic options may include surgical resection, chemotherapy, radiation therapy, hormonal therapy, targeted therapy, or immunotherapy.

Through the continuously increasing understanding of tumor biology, surgical resection of breast cancer has evolved over the last 100 years from Halsted's radical mastectomy to much less extensive and more personalized surgical resections.

Nowadays, decisions regarding the extent of surgical resection for breast cancer take into account tumor biology, disease extent, patient's physiognomy, as well as patient's preferences. The spectrum of surgical procedures may range from partial mastectomy with sentinel lymph node biopsy and adjuvant radiation to double mastectomy sometimes performed with the intent to prevent breast cancer. The advancements in chemotherapy and hormonal therapy have made major radical resections that include pectoralis major muscle or chest wall less common. In addition, breast reconstructive techniques have also significantly improved esthetics and function for many women who undergo surgical resection of breast cancer.

The treatment of breast cancer requires multidisciplinary expertise. Thoracic surgeons are occasionally summoned to assist with the management of breast cancer, mainly in situations when breast cancer invades into the chest wall or if the disease is detected in the internal mammary

Department of Thoracic and Cardiovascular Surgery, The University of Texas MD Anderson Cancer Center, 1515 Holcombe Boulevard, Houston, TX 77030, USA
E-mail address: bsepesi@mdanderson.org

Thorac Surg Clin 27 (2017) 159–163
http://dx.doi.org/10.1016/j.thorsurg.2017.01.009

lymphatic chain (**Figs. 1** and **2**). Both of these scenarios may occur either in the setting of the primarily diagnosed disease or much more commonly in the setting of recurrent disease. Considering the numerous therapeutic options available, close communication among experts from medical and radiation oncology, surgical oncology, and thoracic and plastic surgery is of paramount importance to design the most effective treatment plan that achieves locoregional disease control and preserves the maximal physiologic function and quality of life for patients. Timing and sequence of each therapy are also very important to achieve the best oncologic and functional benefit.

SURGICAL PRINCIPLES FOR THE MANAGEMENT OF BREAST CANCER INVOLVING THE CHEST WALL

The main goal for a thoracic surgeon in the management of the breast cancer invading the chest wall is to provide the best chance for complete (R0) surgical resection to achieve locoregional disease control. Today, situations of large fungating breast cancers eroding through the skin or into the chest wall are rarely faced; therefore, purely palliative resections just to avoid persistent local infection have become less common.

The first therapeutic step in the management of primary breast cancer invading chest wall is usually chemotherapy, often given over a period of months. Chemotherapy for breast cancer has become very effective and has potential to achieve complete pathologic response in up to 60% of patients depending on the tumor characteristics (triple-negative or human growth factor receptor 2-positive breast cancer) and chemotherapeutic regimen used.[2] The effectiveness of systemic therapy in reducing the tumor size or possibly achieving complete response, may create a dilemma for thoracic surgeons about how aggressively to proceed during surgical resection after chemotherapy for previously documented chest wall invasion with breast cancer. In fact, in very highly selected patients who appear to be exceptional responders to chemotherapy and appear to have achieved complete response radiographically, based on negative findings on PET combined with computed tomography (CT) imaging, or based on MRI following chemotherapy, the question of selective elimination of breast cancer surgery arises.[2] Therefore, indications of whether to submit a patient to a potentially morbid chest wall resection should be personalized. The author has taken a selective approach in making this decision. If a patient with breast cancer and chest wall involvement appears to have complete pathologic response to chemotherapy is brought to the operating theatre for the resection of breast tissue, the area of previous tumor site, and pectoralis muscle, biopsies can be sent for frozen section from the area of chest wall involvement. Persistently positive biopsies in the chest wall indicate further resection to achieve complete tumor control. However, if all intraoperative biopsies from the chest wall are negative, the author has elected not to proceed with formal chest wall resection of the previous tumor site in selected cases, if both the imaging and the intraoperative biopsies demonstrated no evidence of viable tumor. This approach, however, requires pathology expertise in differentiating chemotherapy treatment effect and residual tumor on frozen sections. The

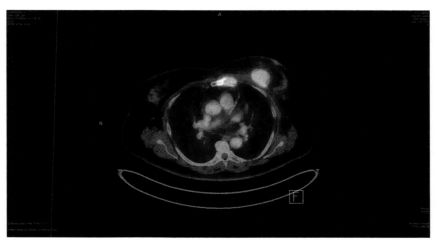

Fig. 1. Breast cancer with spread to internal mammary chain and chest wall.

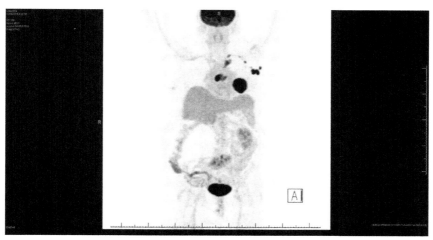

Fig. 2. Primary breast cancer with spread to axillary, supraclavicular, and internal mammary lymph nodes.

judgment of the pathologist as well as the breast and thoracic surgeons in each individual case is of utmost importance in order to achieve the desired outcome. Following chest wall resection for locally invasive breast cancer, adjuvant radiation therapy is indicated; however, this should never be a reason to leave the operating room with a positive microscopic margin.

The more common scenario that requires radical surgical chest wall resection in the setting of breast cancer is in the situation of isolated disease recurrence.[3] Generally, these patients already received multiple cycles of chemotherapy, underwent surgical resection of the primary tumor, and received adjuvant radiation as a component of their initial treatment. This scenario usually precludes further use of radiation therapy as a definitive or adjuvant treatment option (depending on the previous radiation fields, time interval, and tissue tolerance) for isolated locoregional disease recurrence. Operative intervention under such circumstances may be quite complex, depending on the location of the recurrence, and requires multidisciplinary surgery teams and careful treatment planning to achieve optimal outcomes. The expertise of a thoracic surgeon in such a circumstance is very important to assess the anticipated morbidity of the chest wall or sternal resection. Although large multirib or sternal resections are possible,[4] as demonstrated by favorable short-term outcomes following resection of chest wall tumors or locally invasive lung cancer, one must take into consideration whether the large chest wall resection of recurrent breast cancer will achieve improved disease-free or overall survival or merely progression-free survival.

Preoperative workup for chest wall resection of locally advanced or metastatic disease includes detailed medical history and physical examination, documentation of oncologic history, original and most recent staging, understanding of previous treatments, and response to therapeutic measures. Pulmonary and cardiac function tests serve as an additional guide to assess the physiologic reserve. Anatomic studies using either chest CT or chest MRI are necessary for surgical planning. Finally, patients should be presented at multidisciplinary conference to ensure that all available treatment options have been discussed. Surgical plan should be to achieve complete (R0) extirpation of the tumor, and to reconstruct the defect with available prosthetic and/or native tissue grafts to restore both function and cosmetics.

CLINICAL OUTCOMES

Locoregional recurrence following definitive surgical treatment of breast cancer with either total mastectomy or partial mastectomy and adjuvant radiation therapy is associated with variable outcomes with 5-year survival ranging from 18% to 71%.[5] Most of the reports on this topic, however, were limited series that included between 12 and 77 patients, and some of them identified disease-free interval at least 2 years to be associated with favorable outcome.[5]

Approximately 10% to 35% patients with breast cancer may experience either locoregional recurrence alone or in combination with distant metastases. In 2008, Santillan and colleagues[6] reported on outcomes of 28 patients who underwent chest wall resection for recurrent breast cancer involving chest wall or sternum. Interestingly, 57% (16/28) of patients underwent resection for palliation rather than with curative intent. The median disease-free interval before chest wall resection was 4.6 years. Complete R0 resection was achieved in only 71% of patients. There was no perioperative mortality with 21% postoperative morbidity. Overall 5-year survival for the entire study group was 18%. The worst outcomes were observed in patients with triple-negative recurrent breast cancer; there were no survivors at 5 years. Five-year survival of patients with non-triple-negative breast cancer was 39%. Investigators concluded that chest wall resection for recurrent breast cancer can be achieved with acceptable short-term morbidity and low mortality, and that even patients with triple-negative breast cancer should be considered for palliative resection considering the lack of alternative therapies in this patient population.[6]

In 2009, van der Pol and colleagues[3] reported on prognostic factors in 77 curative chest wall resections for isolated breast cancer recurrence. The 5-year overall survival was 25%, and on univariable analysis, investigators found 3 variables to be associated with favorable outcome, namely, interval between original treatment and chest wall resection, administration of chemotherapy for recurrence, and surgical resection of the chest wall less than 150 cm^2 in size. On multivariable analysis, however, only disease-free interval of more than 10 years predicted favorable outcome after chest wall resection, which essentially corroborates with very indolent tumor biology in those patients who recurred more than 10 years after the primary breast cancer treatment.[3]

In a more recent (2013) publication, Shen and colleagues[7] analyzed the "clinical course of breast cancer patients with isolated sternal and full thickness chest wall recurrences treated with and without radical surgery." The study identified 76 patients who were treated for isolated chest wall recurrence from 1992 to 2011 at a large cancer center and attempted to answer the question about the benefit of aggressive surgical resection for recurrent breast cancer. Overall, 44 patients were treated surgically and 32 with other modalities. Five-year survival was not statistically significant between the groups ($P = .52$), although one may argue that nearly 20% difference in 5-year overall survival between the surgical group (30.6%) and nonsurgical group (49.6%) is clinically relevant. This difference, however, is likely mainly due to patient selection because the surgical patients presented with more advanced and biologically aggressive disease, mainly triple-negative breast cancer. On the other hand, the surgical patient cohort included more responders to systemic therapy. An important observation from this study that points to the importance of tumor biology in overall outcome is the fact that the majority

(75%) of patients who were treated nonsurgically experienced chest wall recurrence more than 2 years after the original breast cancer treatment. Among hormone receptor–positive patients, the benefit of surgical resection of recurrence was in improved progression-free survival ($P = .01$), but not in overall survival ($P = .25$). The investigators concluded that systemic therapy should be the initial treatment in a setting of chest wall recurrence, and that consideration for aggressive surgical resection could be offered to patients with hormone-positive disease, patients with good response or stable nonprogressive disease on chemotherapy. Moreover, patients requiring these complex and multidisciplinary operations are likely best served in centers experienced in the complex management of recurrent breast cancer.[7]

Another series of 33 women who underwent aggressive surgical resection of chest wall and other structures, such as subclavian vessels, pericardium, phrenic nerve, of T1 nerve root, for recurrent breast cancer was reported by Levy Faber and colleagues.[8] Although the postoperative morbidity was 36%, there were no perioperative deaths, and at the median follow-up duration of 33 months, median survival was 69 months, with 5-year predicted survival of 63%. Recurrence developed in 13 patients, 12 of which occurred as distant metastases. Five-year disease-free survival was 50%. Investigators concluded that surgical resection of chest wall for recurrent breast cancer should be considered as a treatment option; however, they also astutely pointed out that further studies are needed to identify patients at high risk of distant recurrence.[8]

COMPLICATIONS AND CONCERNS

The rate of complications following chest wall resection and reconstruction for locally invasive breast cancer has not been well documented. However, data regarding complications from the chest wall resection can be extrapolated from other disease processes and published series. Spicer and colleagues[9] have recently reported on pulmonary and infectious complications following chest wall resection and reconstruction for thoracic malignancies involving chest wall. In a series of 427 patients who underwent chest wall resection followed by reconstruction with either flexible or rigid prosthetic material, pulmonary complications occurred in 24% of patients (102/427); infectious complications were uncommon and occurred in 3% of patients (13/427). Interestingly, the type of chest wall reconstruction, whether performed with rigid or flexible material, was not associated with the pulmonary complication rate on multivariable analysis, rather the number of resected ribs (odds ratio [OR] 1.26, confidence interval [CI] 1.00–1.59), or concomitant lung parenchyma resection (lobectomy, OR 3.59, CI 1.62–7.92), were identified as variables associated with perioperative pulmonary morbidity.[9] Investigators concluded that effective chest wall reconstruction can be achieved with either rigid or flexible material, depending on the circumstances. Because randomized data are not available on this topic, bias in terms of the reconstructive material selection used in chest wall reconstructions influenced the results of this study and other previous studies of this topic. It should be noted that many thoracic surgeons tend to reconstruct large chest wall defects with rigid prostheses, such as methyl methacrylate or titanium plates, in combination with other prosthetic or biologic materials or native tissue coverage. However, newer materials such as Gore-Tex or biologic dermal matrixes are very easy to work with and can be sutured to the periphery of the defect under tension, to restore the contour of the chest wall and provide functional stability. Patients who undergo chest wall resection of 1 or 2 ribs generally perform well from the physiologic standpoint, and as long as there is no loss of lung parenchyma, the complication rate of these procedures should be relatively low.

SUMMARY

Surgical resection of the chest wall for locally invasive or recurrent breast cancer dates back more than 100 years to the times of Halsted and colleagues.[10] Since then significant progress has been made in surgical techniques of chest wall resection and reconstruction, thanks to the wider options and availability of reconstructive materials. Most significant progress, however, has been made in the understanding of cancer biology and cancer behavior, and in the development of novel chemotherapeutic agents. Surgical treatment of locally advanced or recurrent breast cancer involving chest wall continues to play a role in the therapeutic armamentarium as part of the multidisciplinary treatment regimen. Patient selection and superb knowledge of the most recent and effective treatment options are necessary to maximize the survival benefit and quality of life of patients affected with breast cancer involving the chest wall.

REFERENCES

1. Available at: http://www.breastcancer.org/symptoms/understand_bc/statistics. Accessed January 10, 2017.
2. van la Parra RF, Kuerer HM. Selective elimination of breast cancer surgery in exceptional responders: historical perspective and current trials. Breast Cancer Res 2016;18(1):28.
3. van der Pol CC, van Geel AN, Menke-Pluymers MB, et al. Prognostic factors in 77 curative chest wall resections for isolated breast cancer recurrence. Ann Surg Oncol 2009;16(12):3414–21.
4. Ahmad U, Yang H, Sima C, et al. Resection of primary and secondary tumors of the sternum: an analysis of prognostic variables. Ann Thorac Surg 2015; 100(1):215–22.
5. D'Aiuto M, Cicalese M, D'Aiuto G, et al. Surgery of the chest wall for involvement by breast cancer. Thorac Surg Clin 2010;20(4):509–17.
6. Santillan AA, Kiluk JV, Cox JM, et al. Outcomes of locoregional recurrence after surgical chest wall resection and reconstruction for breast cancer. Ann Surg Oncol 2008;15(5):1322–9.
7. Shen MC, Massarweh NN, Lari SA, et al. Clinical course of breast cancer patients with isolated sternal and full-thickness chest wall recurrences treated with and without radical surgery. Ann Surg Oncol 2013;20(13):4153–60.
8. Levy Faber D, Fadel E, Kolb F, et al. Outcome of full-thickness chest wall resection for isolated breast cancer recurrence. Eur J Cardiothorac Surg 2013; 44(4):637–42.
9. Spicer JD, Shewale JB, Antonoff MB, et al. The influence of reconstructive technique on perioperative pulmonary and infectious outcomes following chest wall resection. Ann Thorac Surg 2016; 102(5):1653–9.
10. Halsted CP, Benson JR, Jatoi I. A historical account of breast cancer surgery: beware of local recurrence but be not radical. Future Oncol 2014;10(9): 1649–57.

Chest Wall Reconstruction Without Prosthetic Material

Robert E. Merritt, MD

KEYWORDS

- Chest wall resection • Soft tissue reconstruction • Free muscle flap • Pedicled muscle flap

KEY POINTS

- Chest wall tumors often require full-thickness resection of bone, soft tissue, and skin.
- Full-thickness chest wall defects can be covered with soft tissue reconstruction without prosthetic material, such as nonabsorbable mesh or methyl methacrylate.
- Prosthetic mesh or methyl methacrylate requires reoperation and removal in cases complicated by postoperative infection.
- Muscle flaps can be transferred by pedicle muscle transposition or free muscle flap transfer.
- Soft tissue reconstruction should be performed in conjunction with a plastic surgeon.

INTRODUCTION

The most common indication for chest wall resection is a primary neoplasm of the chest wall, such as sarcoma (**Figs. 1–6**). Secondary chest wall tumors, such as metastatic breast cancer, can be completely resected as well with a full-thickness chest wall resection and reconstruction. In addition, direct invasion from a non–small cell lung cancer tumor can also require a full-thickness chest wall resection with reconstruction. A full-thickness chest wall resection often includes ribs, muscle, and skin. After full-thickness resection, a large defect is often present with exposed intrathoracic structures. Prosthetic mesh, such as Marlex, and a more rigid methyl methacrylate mesh have been routinely used to cover the bony chest wall defect after a chest wall resection. Many surgeons think that the prosthetic material stabilizes the chest wall and prevents paradoxic chest wall motion that is seen with flail chest. There are situations when only a soft tissue reconstruction of the chest wall is preferable.

Prosthetic material can become infected and can require reoperation for removal of the infected material. In addition, rigid prosthetic mesh, such as methyl methacrylate, can result in chest wall deformity and chronic pain. Muscle is the soft tissue of choice for coverage of full-thickness chest wall defects. Muscle flaps can be transferred to chest wall defects with either pedicled muscle transposition or free muscle transfer. In most cases, the pedicled muscle transposition is used for soft tissue reconstruction of the chest wall. A multidisciplinary approach with the inclusion of a plastic surgeon will increase the chances of excellent postoperative outcomes for chest wall reconstruction.

INDICATIONS FOR CHEST WALL RESECTION AND RECONSTRUCTION

The indications for chest wall resection with reconstruction include primary and metastatic chest wall tumors (**Box 1**). Most chest wall tumors may involve the ribs, sternum, and soft tissues;

No disclosures.
Division of Thoracic Surgery, The Ohio State University Wexner Medical Center, Doan N-847, 410 West 10th Avenue, Columbus, OH 43210, USA
E-mail address: robert.merritt@osumc.edu

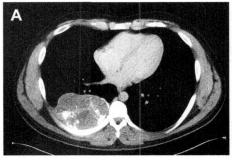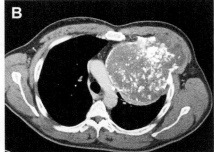

Fig. 1. (*A*) A computed tomographic (CT) scan of the chest demonstrating a synovial cell sarcoma involving the posterior chest wall. (*B*) A CT scan of the chest demonstrating a large chondrosarcoma involving the anterior chest wall.

therefore, a full-thickness resection may be necessary in most cases. The options for chest wall reconstruction include prosthetic and biologic mesh materials, such as Marlex mesh and methyl methacrylate (**Box 2**). Most would agree that full-thickness skeletal defects that are greater than 4 to 5 cm require replacement of the bony chest wall defect with prosthetic material; however, there may be circumstances when prosthetic material cannot be used. Rigid reconstruction of the bony chest wall has become standard because of its effectiveness of stabilizing the thorax. There is a risk of postoperative infection, which would necessitate the removal of the prosthetic material. In cases involving radiation necrosis or a necrotic neoplasm, reconstruction with prosthetic mesh material is not a good option given the risk of infection. In these cases, chest wall reconstruction can be performed with soft tissue reconstruction with a muscle or musculocutaneous flap.

CLASSIFICATION OF MUSCLE FLAPS

The primary goal of tissue muscle flap reconstruction is to provide vascularized tissue coverage of large full-thickness chest wall defects. Muscle flaps are typically described as local or distant. Muscles flaps that are transposed to adjacent locations are considered local flaps. Distant muscle flaps are transposed to more distant sites. A pedicle muscle flap is transferred to a remote site with the blood supply completely intact. A free muscle flap is a distant muscle flap that is connected to remote blood vessels by vascular anastomosis. There is a wide selection of muscle flaps to select from for soft tissue reconstruction of the chest wall (**Box 3**).

LATISSIMUS DORSI MUSCLE FLAP

The latissimus dorsi muscle flap is one of the most commonly used muscle flaps for chest wall reconstruction. This muscle is the largest muscle on the thorax. The muscle is long in length

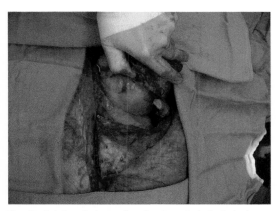

Fig. 2. A lateral view of a chest wall defect during a resection of a large chondrosarcoma. The full-thickness chest wall specimen is being elevated to expose the left thoracic cavity.

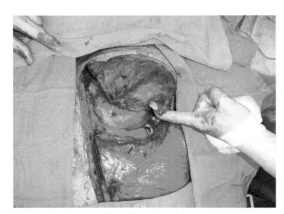

Fig. 3. A chest wall defect involving a hemisternectomy and en bloc chest wall resection.

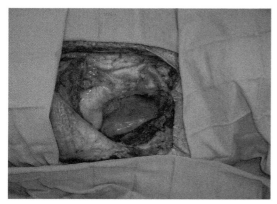

Fig. 4. A full-thickness chest wall defect after a complete chest wall resection. The left lung and mediastinum can be visualized.

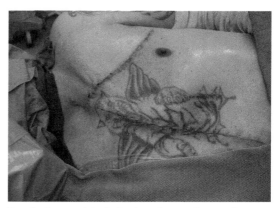

Fig. 6. A completed chest wall resection and reconstruction with a latissimus dorsi muscle flap without prosthetic material.

and has a broad size, which makes it ideal for covering large chest wall defects. The muscle originates from the iliac crest and spine and inserts on the humerus bone. The thoracodorsal artery is the main blood supply, and the thoracodorsal nerve is the primary innervation. The latissimus dorsi muscle can be accessed through a muscle-sparing thoracotomy. The blood supply is located superiorly; therefore, the latissimus flap must be divided inferiorly. The latissimus dorsi muscle can be rotated on its vascular pedicle anteriorly or posteriorly to cover large chest wall defects.[1]

PECTORALIS MAJOR MUSCLE FLAP

The pectoralis major is the second largest muscle of the thorax. The pectoralis major muscle can be used to cover chest wall defects after a resection of the sternum. The pectoralis muscle inserts into the humerus bone and originates from the sternum. The thoracoacromial vessels and perforators from the internal mammary vessels provide the blood supply. The pectoralis major is innervated by the medial pectoral nerve and the lateral anterior thoracic nerve. This muscle can be used an advancement flap by elevating the muscle off of the sternum in the midline. The pectoralis major advancement flap can be used to cover sternal defects after resection of tumors involving the sternum.[2] The pectoralis major muscle can also be used as a rotation flap to cover upper posterior chest wall defects.

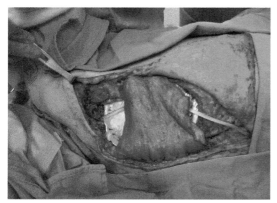

Fig. 5. A pedicled latissimus dorsi muscle flap that has been transposed to cover the full-thickness chest wall defect.

Box 1
Indications for chest wall resection
Primary chest wall tumors
Chondrosarcoma
Osteosarcoma
Desmoid tumor
Synovial cell sarcoma
Rhabdomyosarcoma
Metastatic or direct extension
Non–small cell lung cancer
Breast carcinoma
Renal cell carcinoma
Infection
Sternal wound infection
Radiation necrosis
Osteomyelitis of the chest wall

Box 2
Prosthetic material for chest wall reconstruction

Marlex mesh

Prolene mesh

Vicryl mesh

Methyl methacrylate

Gore-Tex

Bovine pericardium

SERRATUS ANTERIOR MUSCLE FLAP

The serratus anterior muscle can used to cover intrathoracic cavities and the bronchial stump after a lobectomy or pneumonectomy.[3] The serratus anterior inserts on the scapula and originates from ribs 1 to 8. The blood supply is based on the thoracodorsal vessels and the long thoracic vessels. The serratus anterior is usually preserved during a thoracotomy incision. The serratus anterior can be mobilized from the chest wall with cautery while preserving the vascular pedicle superiorly. The transposition of the serratus anterior muscle flap can be performed through the second intercostal place. The serratus anterior muscle can also be used in conjunction with a latissimus dorsi muscle flap.

RECTUS ABDOMINIS MUSCLE FLAP

The rectus abdominis muscle can be used to cover the anterior inferior chest wall defects. The rectus abdominis muscle originates from the pubis bone and costochondral cartilages 5 to 8. The blood supply originates from the internal mammary and inferior epigastric vessels. The rectus abdominis muscle can be used as a simple muscle flap or a myocutaneous flap. The rectus abdominis muscle is prepared based on the internal mammary artery pedicle and can be rotated superiorly to cover an anterior and inferior chest wall defect. The transverse rectus abdominis

---

Box 3
Muscle flaps for chest wall reconstruction

Latissimus dorsi muscle

Pectoralis major muscle

Serratus anterior muscle

Rectus abdominis muscle

External oblique muscle

---

musculocutaneous flap can be used to reconstruct sternal wound defects.[4]

EXTERNAL OBLIQUE MUSCLE FLAP

The external oblique muscle can be transposed to cover chest wall defects of the lower thorax. The blood supply for this muscle flap is the lower thoracic intercostal vessels. The external oblique can be used as a simple muscle flap or a myocutaneous muscle flap.

CLINICAL RESULTS OF CHEST WALL RESECTION WITHOUT PROSTHETIC RECONSTRUCTION

The primary concern after full-thickness chest wall reconstruction is the stability of the thorax. Chest wall reconstruction typically consists of the use of a rigid or nonrigid prosthetic patch to cover the bony defect and a muscle flap to cover the prosthetic material. The use of rigid prosthetic material for chest wall reconstruction has been associated with postoperative pain, infection, and chest wall deformity. The clinical results of chest wall reconstruction without prosthetic material have been reviewed in several reports. Weyant and colleagues[5] reported a series of patients who underwent chest wall reconstruction with and without rigid prosthesis. A total of 53 patients underwent chest wall reconstruction without prosthetic material. The overall 30-day complication rate and mortalities were not significantly different between the patients who underwent chest wall reconstruction with or without prosthetic material. The patients who received rigid or nonrigid prosthetic material had a significantly higher 90-day complication rate and 4% of the patients with prosthetic material underwent prosthesis removal.

Tsukushi and colleagues[6] reported a series of 50 patients who underwent chest wall resection and reconstruction. A total of 18 patients underwent chest wall reconstruction without prosthetic material in which suture stabilization was used to stabilize the chest wall. The complications rate was similar between the patients with and without prosthetic material. Similarly, Hanna and colleagues[7] reported a series of 37 patients who underwent chest wall resection and reconstruction for malignancy. The patients (N = 12) who underwent chest wall reconstruction without prosthetic material did not experience any site infections and did require reoperation for infection. A total of 19% of the patients who underwent chest wall reconstruction with prosthetic material required reoperation for infection. Interestingly, the use of a muscle flap was present in 75% of the cases regardless if prosthetic mesh was used or not. There was no difference in respiratory complications in the patients who underwent chest wall reconstruction with or without prosthetic material.

SUMMARY

Resection of the primary and secondary tumors involving the chest wall often requires reconstruction with prosthetic and soft tissues. The prosthetic material includes rigid mesh, such as methyl methacrylate, and nonrigid mesh, such as Prolene mesh. Soft tissue reconstruction primarily consists of pedicled muscle flaps. There are situations when only a soft tissue reconstruction of the chest wall is preferable. Prosthetic material can become infected and can require reoperation for removal of the infected material. Muscle is the tissue of choice for coverage of full-thickness chest wall defects. Muscle flaps can be transferred to chest wall defects with either pedicle muscle transposition or free muscle transfer. A multidisciplinary approach with the inclusion of a plastic surgeon will increase the chances of excellent postoperative outcomes for chest wall reconstruction.

REFERENCES

1. Bostwick J III, Nahai F, Wallace JG, et al. Sixty latissimus dorsi flaps. Plast Reconstr Surg 1979; 63:31–41.
2. Pairolero PC, Arnold PG. Chondrosarcoma of the manubrium: resection and reconstruction pectoralis major muscle. Mayo Clin Proc 1978;53:54–7.
3. Gleason KG, Miller DL, Johnson CH, et al. Management of the irradiated bronchus after lobectomy for lung cancer. Ann Thorac Surg 2003;76:180–5.
4. Pairolero PC, Arnold PG. Management of recalcitrant median sternotomy wounds. J Thorac Cardiovasc Surg 1984;88:357–64.
5. Weyant MJ, Bains MS, Venkatrman E, et al. Results of chest wall resection and reconstruction with and without rigid prosthesis. Ann Thorac Surg 2006;81: 279–85.
6. Tsukushi S, Nishida Y, Sugiura H, et al. Non-rigid reconstruction of chest wall defects after resection of musculoskeletal tumors. Surg Today 2015;45: 150–5.
7. Hanna WC, Ferri LE, McKendy KM, et al. Reconstruction after major chest wall resection: can rigid fixation be avoided? Surgery 2011;150:590–7.

Surgical Management of the Radiated Chest Wall and Its Complications

Dan J. Raz, MD[a],*, Sharon L. Clancy, MD[b],
Loretta J. Erhunmwunsee, MD[a]

KEYWORDS

- Chest wall • Radiation • Osteonecrosis • Sarcoma • Breast cancer

KEY POINTS

- Radiation to the chest wall is common before resection of tumors.
- History of radiation does not necessarily change the surgical approach of soft tissue coverage needed for reconstruction.
- Osteoradionecrosis can occur after radiation treatment, particularly after high-dose radiation treatment. Radical resection and reconstruction is feasible and can be lifesaving.
- Radiation-induced sarcomas of the chest wall occur most commonly after radiation therapy for breast cancer.
- The most effective treatment is surgical resection. Tumors not amenable to surgical resection are treated with chemotherapy, with low response rates.

Radiation therapy to the chest wall is common, and is most commonly administered for treatment of primary or recurrent breast cancer. Radiation therapy may cause both early and late radiation tissue injury. Radiation therapy causes tissue damage primarily by means of reactive oxygen species–mediated damage to differentiated soft tissue cells, soft tissue progenitor cells, and vascular endothelial cells. These changes lead to fibrosis, an abnormal response to tissue injury, and tissue death.[1] In addition, cytokine and chemokine release after irradiation perpetuate a chronic inflammatory response that can cause ongoing tissue injury. A host of proinflammatory cytokines, including interleukin (IL)-1, IL-6, transforming growth factor beta, and tumor necrosis factor alpha, contribute to the chronic inflammation and tissue damage observed after radiation therapy.[1–4]

A spectrum of chest wall injury can be seen after radiation treatment. Skin toxicity, including hyperpigmentation, telangiectasias, and dryness, is common.[5,6] Soft tissue edema and minor fat necrosis are fairly common. Rib fractures can occur and may lead to acute and chronic pain. Symptomatic chest wall tissue injury with impending or early skin ulceration may benefit from hyperbaric oxygen treatment (Hbo_2).[7,8] Hbo_2 involves administration of pure oxygen in a pressurized chamber, typically greater than 2 atm, dosed as daily or twice-daily sessions. Hbo_2 increases the partial pressure of oxygen in the soft tissues and has been shown to speed healing of radiation-induced injury. The most common use of Hbo_2 for treatment of radiation-associated tissue injury is for osteoradionecrosis of the mandible in the setting of head and neck cancer; however, Hbo_2

Disclosure: D.J. Raz is a consultant for Cireca LLC, and has received grant funding from Merck; S.L. Clancy and L.J. Erhunmwunsee have nothing to disclose.
[a] Division of Thoracic Surgery, City of Hope, MOB 2001B, 1500 East Duarte Road, Duarte, CA 91010, USA;
[b] Division of Plastic Surgery, City of Hope, MOB 2001B, 1500 East Duarte Road, Duarte, CA 91010, USA
* Corresponding author.
E-mail address: draz@coh.org

Thorac Surg Clin 27 (2017) 171–179
http://dx.doi.org/10.1016/j.thorsurg.2017.01.011

treatment of chest wall wounds has also been used with some reported success.[7,9,10]

At the other end of the spectrum of radiation-induced soft tissue injury are severe osteoradionecrosis and radiation-induced sarcoma.[5,11] Osteoradionecrosis presents with ulceration and sometimes extensive soft tissue changes. When left untreated, full-thickness necrosis ensues and superimposed infection can occur. Soft tissue biopsy is recommended to rule out recurrent breast cancer, because this may change the treatment approach with regard to determining the goals of surgery and use of preoperative therapies. Radiation-induced sarcomas should similarly be biopsied with core needle biopsy to exclude recurrent breast cancer.

This article focuses on surgical resection of the chest wall after radiation therapy. It concentrates mainly on treatment of osteoradionecrosis and radiation-induced sarcomas, although it briefly discusses surgical resection of recurrent cancers in the setting of radiation therapy.

SURGICAL RESECTION OF THE IRRADIATED CHEST WALL

In addition to surgical resection for osteonecrosis and radiation-induced sarcoma (discussed later), surgical resection of recurrent breast and chest wall sarcoma after radiation therapy is sometimes necessary.[12–14] Locoregional recurrence of breast cancer in the chest wall occurs in approximately 9% of patients undergoing breast conservation therapy.[14] Multimodality treatment, including chemotherapy, radiation, and surgery, is typically used. Although there is some controversy regarding the benefit of surgery compared with systemic therapy and radiation therapy in estrogen receptor–negative breast cancer, surgical resection is often performed after radiation therapy has already been administered to the chest wall. In general, resection margins should encompass all skin with radiation changes to ensure proper wound healing. Surgical margins should be appropriately wide. Although the authors recommend and routinely use intraoperative frozen section analysis, margin determination can be challenging at bony margins where frozen section is not possible. In addition, frozen section analysis of breast cancer at soft tissue margins can sometimes miss infiltrating breast cancer cells that are identified on permanent pathology.[15–17] Reconstruction of the chest wall is described elsewhere. Soft tissue coverage should factor in the size of the defect, the radiation field, and the quality of the soft tissue at any potential flap vascular pedicle. Rotational myocutaneous flaps, such as latissimus dorsi flaps, are commonly used but close attention should be directed to whether the vascular pedicle was included in the radiation field and, if so, whether the vessels are patent and what the quality of the soft tissue surrounding those vessels is.[18] These considerations can affect the blood flow to the flap after reconstruction, even when vessels are patent, through kinking of the pedicle when rotated through fibrotic tissue. Similarly, free flaps should be implanted into vessels free of radiation whenever possible. Use of the omentum, which is tunneled subcutaneously, provides excellent soft tissue coverage in an irradiated field and is covered with skin grafting. The downsides of omental flaps are the need for laparotomy (or laparoscopic harvest), risk of symptomatic ventral hernia, and inferior cosmetic result. In addition, the omentum may not provide sufficient coverage in very thin patients. Selection of coverage should be individualized based on the size of the defect, extent of radiation changes, and body habitus.[19]

OSTEONECROSIS OF THE CHEST WALL

Aside from skin changes and soft tissue edema, chest wall necrosis is rare with standard doses of radiation therapy (typically 4000–5000 cGy). Although there is not much evidence on the factors contributing to chest wall osteoradionecrosis, delivery of high-dose radiation, either planned or unplanned, because of incorrect planning, dose calculation, or machine calculation, is likely to be responsible.[20] Patients typically present with slowly worsening skin ulceration and full-thickness necrosis that involves pathologic rib fractures, which cause discomfort and chest wall instability. Tissue necrosis often progresses with time because of a combination of ongoing microvascular compromise, inflammation, and infection. Localized infection in the skin, soft tissue, and bone is common because of the loss of the normal skin barrier and compromised microvascular circulation, which prevents an effective immune response. When allowed to progress without treatment, loss of necrotic soft tissue and ribs exposes the thoracic viscera, which results in empyema. Both soft tissue infection and empyema may result in septicemia, which may be fatal if left untreated. Quality of life is poor because of fatigue from chronic wound infection, the foul smell that often accompanies infection, and body image issues related to the nature of the wound.

It is important to biopsy the edges of the wound to rule out recurrent cancer. At times, it can be difficult to distinguish osteoradionecrosis from recurrent cancer, and both may be present.

Imaging with chest computed tomography (CT) and PET/CT is important to evaluate for systemic disease; however, imaging is not diagnostic to distinguish between these 2 entities. Although both recurrent disease and osteoradionecrosis are typically treated surgically, recurrent breast cancer in the chest wall is associated with poor prognosis and systemic therapy before surgical resection may be indicated. Moreover, surgical margins should be wider when recurrent chest wall disease is present.

The primary goals of surgical treatment of osteoradionecrosis are to eliminate infection, to excise all damaged tissue, and to provide stability to the chest wall during reconstruction. When infection of ulcerated skin is present, a combination of systemic antibiotic therapy, localized wound debridement, and vacuum-assisted closure (VAC) therapy (KCI, San Antonio, TX) is often indicated. VAC therapy accelerates wound healing by applying negative pressure, removing edema fluid and bacteria. This process improves resolution of infection and decreases time to formation of granulation tissue.[21]

It is important to reduce the bacterial load of the soft tissue as much as possible before definitive surgical resection, because prosthetic chest wall reconstruction provides the most effective stabilization of the chest wall. The extent of debridement varies by the extent of wet necrosis. Options for debridement include mechanical (surgical) debridement, enzymatic debridement, and maggot debridement therapy (MDT). For extensive chest wall wounds, the authors have used MDT with excellent results.[22] Enzymatic debridement, such as collagenase SANTYL ointment, typically must be used in combination with mechanical debridement and is not very effective for most chest wall wounds on its own.

Surgical resection should involve a plastic reconstructive surgeon for soft tissue coverage. As previously mentioned, the use of rotational myocutaneous flap, most often a latissimus dorsi flap, is based on the field of radiation, the quality of the vascular bundle supplying the flap, the quality of the tissues surrounding the vascular bundle, the patient's body habitus, and the size and location of the defect. Omental flap is an excellent and versatile option but it involves intra-abdominal surgery and the cosmetic outcome may be less appealing compared with myocutaneous flap coverage.

Surgical resection should encompass all skin and soft tissue that grossly appears to be compromised by radiation therapy. Resection of chest wall should continue to healthy bleeding tissues. Resection of underlying lung is occasionally necessary when it is adherent to the chest wall

because of radiation-associated adhesions. Options for chest wall resection are discussed elsewhere in detail, but include no reconstruction, prosthetic reconstruction, and biological reconstruction. The authors favor reconstruction for all anterior chest wall defects, except in small chest wall defects involving 1 rib or short segments of 2 ribs. Reconstruction provides improved chest wall stability and improves quality of life. Rigid prosthetic chest wall reconstructions provide the best mechanical support for the chest wall. The authors most commonly use Marlex mesh with methyl methacrylate patch because these materials create a reconstruction that provides rigid reconstruction that can be shaped or molded as needed and is inexpensive. Others use a combination of rib plating devices (osteosynthesis) and mesh, although this approach is substantially more expensive. One of the risks of implanting a prosthetic device is infection, and in a contaminated wound these risks may be substantially higher. The use of biological meshes decreases the risk of infection but provides inferior mechanical support compared with rigid prosthetic reconstruction. Several biological meshes are available, but most are thin and do not provide the stability needed in chest wall reconstruction. To our knowledge, SurgiMend bovine acellular matrix is the thickest biological patch (4-mm thickness) available for reconstruction. The authors have used this patch for chest wall reconstruction in the setting of infection with good results.

Here this article presents a case of osteoradionecrosis as an example of some of the challenges associated with treatment of this problem.

Case Presentation

A 48-year-old woman was diagnosed with ER+/PR+/Her2+ left breast cancer 4 years before presentation. She delayed her treatment and opted to receive high-dose radiation treatment to the breast and chest wall over a 7-month period several years later. Soon after completion of her treatment, she developed dyspnea and was found to have pulmonary metastases. She was started on systemic chemotherapy followed by tamoxifen. At that time, she developed a chronic chest wall wound, which was periodically treated with oral antibiotics and the patient required narcotics for pain control. The wound became progressively deeper, purulent, and malodorous and at that point she transferred her care to our institution. The ulceration was approximately 14 × 16 cm with exposed necrotic ribs visible and extensive yellow necrotic fibrinous material lining the wound (**Figs. 1** and **2**). The edges of the wound were darkened and

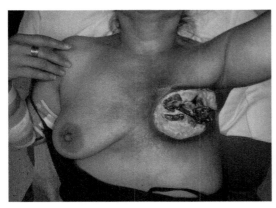

Fig. 1. Chest wall ulceration showing extensive fibrinous exudate, exposed ribs, and radiation changes to the skin surrounding the ulceration.

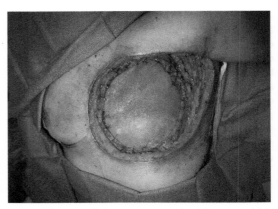

Fig. 3. Chest wall is reconstructed with 4-mm-thick SurgiMend and secured to surrounding ribs and sternum with interrupted 0-Prolene mattress sutures.

thickened and extended about 3 cm in all directions. Punch biopsy of adjacent skin showed no evidence of carcinoma. A peripherally inserted central catheter line and antibiotic therapy were initiated, and MDT was initiated by the dermatology service. Trastuzumab (Herceptin) was initiated by the treating oncologist for the metastatic disease. After 6 weeks of intravenous antibiotics and maggot therapy, the patient underwent surgical resection. The ulcerated portion of the chest wall and all skin changes were excised. Portions of ribs 2 to 5 and a portion of the sternum were resected. A wedge resection of the left upper lobe was also performed because of adherence to the chest wall (**Fig. 3**). The chest wall was reconstructed with 4-mm-thick SurgiMend (**Fig. 4**). The plastic surgery service then performed latissimus dorsi and serratus anterior muscle flaps with split-thickness skin grafting to cover the soft tissue

defect (**Fig. 5**). However, the latissimus dorsi muscle flap developed partial necrosis, and the patient was taken back to the operating room and an omental flap was harvested via laparotomy and transposed subcutaneously to cover the defect (**Fig. 6**). Split-thickness skin graft was harvested to cover the omental flap. The patient then had an uneventful recovery (**Fig. 7**). She is alive with stable disease more than 2 years after her operation.

RADIATION-INDUCED SOFT TISSUE AND BONE CANCERS OF THE CHEST WALL

Sarcomas make up approximately 1% of all cancers. Different factors have been linked to their formation, including viruses, genetic predisposition, chronic edema, chemotherapy, and radiation therapy. Ionizing radiation exposure is only linked to 3% to 5% of all sarcomas.[23,24] Seventy percent of these tumors are soft tissue tumors, whereas

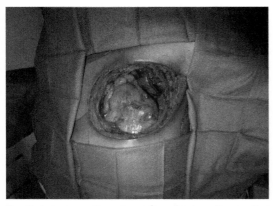

Fig. 2. Intraoperative view after chest wall resection showing bleeding soft tissue wound edges. The heart and left lung are visible in the base of the wound. The soft tissue resection extended into the axilla.

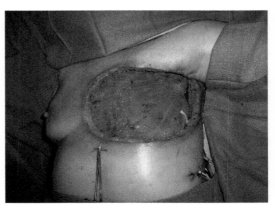

Fig. 4. Intraoperative view after latissimus dorsi and serratus anterior rotational flaps are secured for soft tissue coverage.

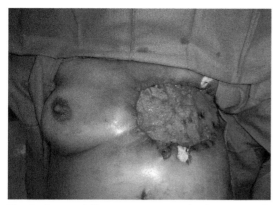

Fig. 5. Omental flap was transposed subcutaneously after latissimus dorsi flap necrosis.

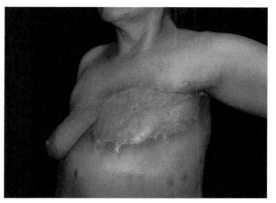

Fig. 7. Three-month postoperative image showing healed skin graft over omental reconstruction.

the other 30% develop in bone.[24] Radiation-induced sarcomas (RISs) can be of a variety of histologies, the most frequent being (1) undifferentiated pleomorphic sarcoma, previously termed malignant fibrous histiocytoma[25]; and (2) angiosarcoma, primarily occurring among women treated with external radiation therapy for breast cancer.[24] The most common type of radiotherapy (RT)-induced bone sarcoma is osteosarcoma.[23]

The frequency of RIS is less than 1%,[4] although the incidence is slightly more than 1% in children previously treated with radiation.[26] RISs are primarily a complication of high-dose therapy, and are rarely seen after low doses.[27] Tucker and colleagues[28] found that patients with a history of radiation therapy had a 2.7-fold increased risk and a sharp dose-response gradient reaching a 40-fold risk after doses to the bone of more than 6000 rad.

RISs of the chest wall are typically related to radiation for breast cancer or Hodgkin disease but may occur secondary to lung cancer radiation as well.[25,29–31] In their prospective, descriptive study,

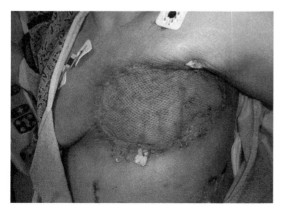

Fig. 6. Postoperative view showing omental flap covered with a split-thickness skin graft harvested from the thigh.

Penel and colleagues[32] evaluated 658 patients with soft tissue sarcomas. Ten of the 22 (45%) RISs observed were in patients with breast cancer, and the next most frequent primary cancer was non-Hodgkin lymphoma (4 patients; 18%). The mean interval from the first cancer treatment to diagnosis of RIS was about 10 years. Souba and colleagues[25] retrospectively evaluated 16 patients who presented with sarcomas of the chest wall at a site where a prior malignancy had been irradiated. Ten (63%) of the 16 patients had prior breast cancer, whereas 4 (25%) had Hodgkin disease. The latency period between irradiation and the development of the chest wall sarcoma ranged from 5 to 28 years, with a mean of 13 years. Among these 16 cases, 6 were osteosarcomas (4 sternal and 2 clavicular/scapular) and 7 were malignant fibrous histiocytomas (MFHs) (1 sternal, 2 lateral chest wall, and 4 supraclavicular). There was 1 lateral chest wall malignant mesenchymoma. The mean survival of patients after diagnosis of the secondary tumor was 13.5 months.

Typically, RISs occur near the edge of the radiation field, which is where the radiation dose can be large enough to cause genetic damage but not so great that the cells are killed. It is unclear whether there is a lower risk with very high doses or whether there is a plateau in risk.[27] Sarcoma formation in Japanese atomic bomb survivors suggests that there is increased risk of RT-induced sarcomas even with low doses of ionizing radiation.[33,34] The addition of chemotherapy, especially alkylating agents, may potentiate the effect of previous radiation therapy.[28] Tucker and colleagues[28] evaluated more than 9700 survivors of childhood cancers. There were 64 cases of bone sarcoma in these survivors. These cases were matched to patients who had not developed a sarcoma. After adjusting for RT, treatment with alkylating agents was linked to bone cancer. Other studies also link the use of alkylating chemotherapy to higher rates of secondary sarcomas in children whose primary tumors were treated with radiation.[35,36] However, these data are not as clear in adult patients.

Diagnosis

Many patients with RIS have a delay in diagnosis because of nonspecific symptoms and radiation changes and fibrosis that may make palpation of a mass difficult. In those who have undergone prior radiation and have new bone or soft tissue pain and/or a new mass, appropriate imaging should be performed. A radiograph is typically the first imaging performed, although cross-sectional imaging is necessary to properly diagnose and characterize the mass.

Patients with breast or breast skin changes are likely to undergo mammography, whereas most others have CT or MRI. MRI is preferred by some clinicians because of its ability to delineate soft tissue structures. The National Comprehensive Cancer Network suggests that PET may be useful in staging, prognostication, grading, and determining response to chemotherapy.[37] A recent meta-analysis suggests that PET may be a promising tool to help predict survival outcomes of patients with bone and soft tissue sarcomas.[38]

It is essential that suspected RISs are biopsied for diagnosis and grading. Core needle biopsies are preferred to fine-needle aspiration whenever feasible.[39] Open diagnostic biopsy is rarely required but may be useful if the other techniques are not feasible. It is imperative that the biopsy site, no matter the technique, be completely removed at the time of resection.

Diagnostic Criteria

Not all sarcomas that arise after prior radiation are secondary to radiation exposure. Some of these sarcomas are sporadic even if they arise in an irradiated field. The following criteria for determination of whether a sarcoma is secondary to radiation exposure were originally proposed by Cahan and colleagues[40] in 1948 and later revised by Murray and colleagues[41]:

1. Radiation must have been given previously and the sarcoma that subsequently developed must have arisen in the area included within the 5% isodose line.
2. There must be no evidence that the sarcoma was present before onset of radiation.
3. Any sarcoma associated with radiation requires histologic confirmation and must be of different histology than the primary tumor.

There is typically a latency period between the treatment of the primary tumor and the appearance of the radiation-induced sarcoma. The usual length of this period is debated. In 1948, Cahan and colleagues[40] proposed a 5-year latency period. Others investigators have suggested a shorter latency period, from as little as 6 months to 4 years.[42–44]

Staging

Staging for both primary and secondary sarcomas of the chest wall is the same. Tumors are characterized by grade and local extension. The American Joint Committee on Cancer (AJCC) seventh edition staging system for soft tissue sarcoma is based on the TNM (tumor, node, metastasis) system. For the T (primary tumor) component, tumors less than 5 cm are T1, whereas tumors larger than 5 cm are T2. Both T1 and T2 lesions are then divided into A and B sections based on whether the tumor is superficial (located above the superficial fascia) or not. N is a based on regional lymph nodes. N1 describes regional lymph node metastasis. If there are nodal metastases, the patient is stage III. M1 suggests distant metastasis. Histologic grades are 1 to 3. The anatomic stage is based on T, N, M, and grade.[37] For bone cancer the T stage is divided at the 8-cm mark. T1 occurs when the primary tumor is up to 8 cm and T2 when greater than 8 cm. T3 is noted if the tumor is discontinuous with the primary bone site. N1 again notes regional lymph node metastasis. Distant metastasis is noted as M1. M1a denotes metastasis to the lungs. M1b describes metastasis to other sides. G1 is well differentiated or low grade. G2 is moderately differentiated, whereas G3 is poorly differentiated, and G4 is undifferentiated.[37] The lung is the predominant site of metastases for both soft tissue and bone sarcomas, whether primary or radiation associated. CT of the chest is typically performed to detect pulmonary metastases in patients with either a soft tissue or bone sarcoma. PET or bone scan is recommended for patients with a bone sarcoma.

Prognosis

Gladdy and colleagues[45] evaluated 130 patients with primary radiation-associated soft tissue sarcomas. These patients were matched with patients with sporadic MFH. The radiation-associated tumors were frequently high grade (83%) and were associated with worse 5-year disease-specific survival (44%) than sporadic tumors (66%). In addition, histologic type, margin status, and tumor size were the most important independent predictors of survival in patients with radiation-associated sarcomas.

Bjerkehagen and colleagues[46] similarly performed a case-control study comparing the survival of radiation-induced sarcoma patients (98 patients) with that of patients with sporadic sarcoma (239 patients with high-grade malignant sarcomas). The 5-year survival of patients with RIS was 32%, whereas it was 51% for those with sporadic high-grade malignant sarcomas ($P>.001$). Female gender, central tumor site, and incomplete surgical remission were significantly more frequent among the patients with RIS than in controls. Incomplete surgical remission, metastases at presentation, microscopic tumor necrosis, and central tumor site were also significant adverse prognostic factors.

Treatment

Surgery with wide local resection is the main treatment of RIS of the chest wall. Chapelier and colleagues[31] evaluated 15 patients who underwent radical resection of RIS of the chest wall. The surgical patients had no evidence of extrathoracic metastases. They were worked up with bronchoscopy, arterial blood gas, and spirometry. Selective arteriography was used to assess the blood supply of available muscle or musculocutaneous flaps in those with sternal and anterolateral tumors. Ten of the patients had a history of breast cancer and 5 of Hodgkin disease. The median delivered radiation dose to the primary tumor site was 45 Gy and the median interval between RT and diagnosis of sarcoma was 14 years. There were 7 tumors located on the sternum, 3 on the lateral chest wall, and 5 in the thoracic outlet. The investigators performed 4 sternectomies, 3 partial sternectomies, 3 lateral chest wall resections, and 5 resections of tumors in the thoracic outlet. Local recurrence occurred in 7 patients after a median interval of 10 months, 4 underwent a repeat resection, and 3 died. They had an overall 5-year survival of 48% and a 5-year disease-free survival of 27%. The study revealed the possibility of long-term survival with surgical resection of RIS and therefore the investigators suggest that radical surgical resection is an integral part of the treatment of these tumors.

Operative Technique

Chapelier and colleagues[31] perform aggressive wide local resection of invaded skin, subcutaneous tissue, irradiated tissues, and scars, including a margin of at least 4 cm of normal surrounding tissue. Resection of sternal tumors are started over the costal margins and include 3 cm of free ribs on each side but spare the unaffected lateral part of the pectoralis major muscles. A total sternectomy is undertaken for tumors located over the midsternum and for large tumors of the manubrium, including the internal third of the clavicles. For lateral chest wall tumors, the free margins of the resection are 1 normal rib above and 1 below. The pleural cavity is entered far away from any chest wall involvement. Lung and involved mediastinal structures are resected en bloc. Tumors invading the thoracic outlet require a transcervical thoracic approach for radical resection of involved structures, including an L-shaped cervicotomy extending into the deltopectoral groove and resection of the internal half of the clavicle. Microscopic evaluation of the margins by frozen section is routinely performed. The investigators resect en bloc any resectable involved structure, such as lung, mediastinal vessel, and pericardium. They suggest that involvement of subclavian and brachiocephalic veins be managed by ligation and excision, whereas involvement of the superior vena cava and the subclavian artery requires prosthetic revascularization with polytetrafluoroethylene.

Chapelier and colleagues[31] go on to recommend resection of T1 or C8 nerve roots or the lower trunk of the brachial plexus to obtain tumor-free margins. They recommend stabilization of the chest wall only in patients with large anterior and anterolateral defects, especially after total sternectomy. Soft tissue reconstruction after radical resection of RIS should be accomplished using a muscle or musculocutaneous flap, necessitating the consultation of a plastics and reconstruction surgeon.

Adjuvant Therapy

Full-dose radiation treatment of RIS is usually not performed because of the prior exposure and increased risk of complications. Hyperfractionated RT with small daily doses, intensity-modulated RT protons, and brachytherapy are possible local control options if surgery is not possible or margins are not clear, but the increased risk of repeat radiation must be measured against its potential benefit. Hyperthermia enhances the effect of radiation and/or chemotherapy and is used frequently to boost the low maximally permitted RT dose in the treatment of recurrences in previously irradiated areas. de Jong and colleagues[47] evaluated the role of reirradiation and hypothermia in the treatment of RIS in the thoracic region. They gave this regimen to 13 patients who had unresectable disease and to 3 patients after surgical resection of the RIS. Their RT consisted of 32 Gy in 8 fractions given twice per week over a period of 4 weeks or 36 Gy in 12 fractions given 4 times per week. Heat was induced electromagnetically by using externally applied, flexible-contact microstrip applicators operating at 434 MHz. For all patients, temperatures were measured on the skin. The target temperature was between 41°C and 43°C for 1 hour. There was a 75% response rate. Six patients remained free of local failure until death or last follow-up. The investigators concluded that reirradiation and hyperthermia for RIS in the thoracic region is feasible because it is associated with a high response rate and the possibility of durable local control. Adjuvant chemotherapy is typically advocated because of the poor prognosis of RIS. However, there are few primary data addressing the benefit in RIS. Lagrange and colleagues[48] compared the survival of 80 patients with RIS. Twenty-eight patients underwent surgery only, 18 patients underwent surgery and chemotherapy, 15 patients were only treated with chemotherapy, and 14 with just RT. Overall survival rates at 2 and 5 years, respectively, were 69% and 39% for patients treated with surgery, 10% and 0% for those treated with chemotherapy, and 52% and 35% for those treated with surgery and chemotherapy ($P = .001$). The 2-year and 5-year rates for survival without recurrence were 54% and 32%, respectively. The lack of convincing data associated with treatment of RIS with chemotherapy suggests that decisions about chemotherapy must be individualized.

In conclusion, RIS of the chest wall occurs very infrequently after treatment of breast or lung cancer, Hodgkin lymphoma, and other tumor types. The interval to diagnosis is typically greater than a decade after the primary treatment. These tumors are frequently high grade and associated with poor prognosis. Radical resection with wide tumor-free margins is the only proven treatment with a long survival and potential cure. The role of chemotherapy and radiation is unclear and their use should be individualized.

REFERENCES

1. Kim JH, Jenrow KA, Brown SL. Mechanisms of radiation-induced normal tissue toxicity and implications for future clinical trials. Radiat Oncol J 2014; 32(3):103–15.

2. Martin M, Lefaix J, Delanian S. TGF-beta1 and radiation fibrosis: a master switch and a specific therapeutic target? Int J Radiat Oncol Biol Phys 2000; 47(2):277–90.

3. Janko M, Ontiveros F, Fitzgerald TJ, et al. IL-1 generated subsequent to radiation-induced tissue injury contributes to the pathogenesis of radiodermatitis. Radiat Res 2012;178(3):166–72.

4. Nawroth I, Alsner J, Behlke MA, et al. Intraperitoneal administration of chitosan/DsiRNA nanoparticles targeting TNFalpha prevents radiation-induced fibrosis. Radiother Oncol 2010;97(1):143–8.

5. Yi A, Kim HH, Shin HJ, et al. Radiation-induced complications after breast cancer radiation therapy: a pictorial review of multimodality imaging findings. Korean J Radiol 2009;10(5):496–507.

6. Johansson S, Svensson H, Denekamp J. Dose response and latency for radiation-induced fibrosis, edema, and neuropathy in breast cancer patients. Int J Radiat Oncol Biol Phys 2002;52(5):1207–19.

7. Hart GB, Mainous EG. The treatment of radiation necrosis with hyperbaric oxygen (OHP). Cancer 1976; 37(6):2580–5.

8. Feldmeier JJ. Hyperbaric oxygen for delayed radiation injuries. Undersea Hyperb Med 2004;31(1): 133–45.

9. Carl UM, Feldmeier JJ, Schmitt G, et al. Hyperbaric oxygen therapy for late sequelae in women receiving radiation after breast-conserving surgery. Int J Radiat Oncol Biol Phys 2001;49(4):1029–31.

10. Carl UM, Hartmann KA. Hyperbaric oxygen treatment for symptomatic breast edema after radiation therapy. Undersea Hyperb Med 1998;25(4):233–4.

11. Granick MS, Larson DL, Solomon MP. Radiation-related wounds of the chest wall. Clin Plast Surg 1993;20(3):559–71.

12. Wouters MW, van Geel AN, Nieuwenhuis L, et al. Outcome after surgical resections of recurrent chest wall sarcomas. J Clin Oncol 2008;26(31): 5113–8.

13. David EA, Marshall MB. Review of chest wall tumors: a diagnostic, therapeutic, and reconstructive challenge. Semin Plast Surg 2011;25(1):16–24.

14. van der Pol CC, van Geel AN, Menke-Pluymers MB, et al. Prognostic factors in 77 curative chest wall resections for isolated breast cancer recurrence. Ann Surg Oncol 2009;16(12):3414–21.

15. Balch GC, Mithani SK, Simpson JF, et al. Accuracy of intraoperative gross examination of surgical margin status in women undergoing partial mastectomy for breast malignancy. Am Surg 2005;71(1): 22–7 [discussion: 27–8].

16. Riedl O, Fitzal F, Mader N, et al. Intraoperative frozen section analysis for breast-conserving therapy in 1016 patients with breast cancer. Eur J Surg Oncol 2009;35(3):264–70.

17. Weber WP, Engelberger S, Viehl CT, et al. Accuracy of frozen section analysis versus specimen radiography during breast-conserving surgery for nonpalpable lesions. World J Surg 2008;32(12): 2599–606.

18. Makboul M, Salama Ayyad MA. Is myocutaneous flap alone sufficient for reconstruction of chest wall osteoradionecrosis? Interact Cardiovasc Thorac Surg 2012;15(3):447–51.

19. Matros E, Disa JJ. Uncommon flaps for chest wall reconstruction. Semin Plast Surg 2011;25(1):55–9.

20. Larson DL, McMurtrey MJ, Howe HJ, et al. Major chest wall reconstruction after chest wall irradiation. Cancer 1982;49(6):1286–93.

21. Siegel HJ, Long JL, Watson KM, et al. Vacuum-assisted closure for radiation-associated wound complications. J Surg Oncol 2007;96(7):575–82.

22. Sun X, Jiang K, Chen J, et al. A systematic review of maggot debridement therapy for chronically infected wounds and ulcers. Int J Infect Dis 2014;25:32–7.

23. Bjerkehagen B, Smeland S, Walberg L, et al. Radiation-induced sarcoma: 25-year experience from the Norwegian Radium Hospital. Acta Oncol 2008; 47(8):1475–82.

24. Brady MS, Gaynor JJ, Brennan MF. Radiation-associated sarcoma of bone and soft tissue. Arch Surg 1992;127(12):1379–85.

25. Souba WW, McKenna RJ Jr, Meis J, et al. Radiation-induced sarcomas of the chest wall. Cancer 1986; 57(3):610–5.

26. Nguyen F, Rubino C, Guerin S, et al. Risk of a second malignant neoplasm after cancer in childhood treated with radiotherapy: correlation with the integral dose restricted to the irradiated fields. Int J Radiat Oncol Biol Phys 2008;70(3):908–15.

27. Berrington de Gonzalez A, Gilbert E, Curtis R, et al. Second solid cancers after radiation therapy: a systematic review of the epidemiologic studies of the radiation dose-response relationship. Int J Radiat Oncol Biol Phys 2013;86(2):224–33.

28. Tucker MA, D'Angio GJ, Boice JD Jr, et al. Bone sarcomas linked to radiotherapy and chemotherapy in children. N Engl J Med 1987;317(10):588–93.

29. Ninomiya H, Miyoshi T, Shirakusa T, et al. Postradiation sarcoma of the chest wall: report of two cases. Surg Today 2006;36(12):1101–4.

30. Mayer R, Aigner C, Stranzl H, et al. Radiation-induced osteosarcoma of the chest wall. Breast J 2002;8(5):320–2.

31. Chapelier AR, Bacha EA, de Montpreville VT, et al. Radical resection of radiation-induced sarcoma of the chest wall: report of 15 cases. Ann Thorac Surg 1997;63(1):214–9.

32. Penel N, Grosjean J, Robin YM, et al. Frequency of certain established risk factors in soft tissue sarcomas in adults: a prospective descriptive study of 658 cases. Sarcoma 2008;2008:459386.

33. Samartzis D, Nishi N, Cologne J, et al. Ionizing radiation exposure and the development of soft-tissue sarcomas in atomic-bomb survivors. J Bone Joint Surg Am 2013;95(3):222–9.

34. Samartzis D, Nishi N, Hayashi M, et al. Exposure to ionizing radiation and development of bone sarcoma: new insights based on atomic-bomb survivors of Hiroshima and Nagasaki. J Bone Joint Surg Am 2011;93(11):1008–15.

35. Henderson TO, Rajaraman P, Stovall M, et al. Risk factors associated with secondary sarcomas in childhood cancer survivors: a report from the Childhood Cancer Survivor Study. Int J Radiat Oncol Biol Phys 2012;84(1):224–30.

36. Menu-Branthomme A, Rubino C, Shamsaldin A, et al. Radiation dose, chemotherapy and risk of soft tissue sarcoma after solid tumours during childhood. Int J Cancer 2004;110(1):87–93.

37. Von Mehren M, Randall RL, Benjamin RS. Soft Tissue Sarcoma, Version 2.2016, NCCN Clinical Practice Guidelines in Oncology. J Natl Compr Canc Netw 2016;14(6):758–86.

38. Li YJ, Dai YL, Cheng YS, et al. Positron emission tomography (18)F-fluorodeoxyglucose uptake and prognosis in patients with bone and soft tissue sarcoma: a meta-analysis. Eur J Surg Oncol 2016; 42(8):1103–14.

39. Domanski HA. Fine-needle aspiration cytology of soft tissue lesions: diagnostic challenges. Diagn Cytopathol 2007;35(12):768–73.

40. Cahan WG, Woodard HQ, Higinbotham NL, et al. Sarcoma arising in irradiated bone; report of 11 cases. Cancer 1948;1(1):3–29.

41. Murray EM, Werner D, Greeff EA, et al. Postradiation sarcomas: 20 cases and a literature review. Int J Radiat Oncol Biol Phys 1999;45(4):951–61.

42. Arlen M, Higinbotham NL, Huvos AG, et al. Radiation-induced sarcoma of bone. Cancer 1971;28(5): 1087–99.

43. Laskin WB, Silverman TA, Enzinger FM. Postradiation soft tissue sarcomas. An analysis of 53 cases. Cancer 1988;62(11):2330–40.

44. Cha C, Antonescu CR, Quan ML, et al. Long-term results with resection of radiation-induced soft tissue sarcomas. Ann Surg 2004;239(6):903–9 [discussion: 909–10].

45. Gladdy RA, Qin LX, Moraco N, et al. Do radiation-associated soft tissue sarcomas have the same prognosis as sporadic soft tissue sarcomas? J Clin Oncol 2010;28(12):2064–9.

46. Bjerkehagen B, Smastuen MC, Hall KS, et al. Why do patients with radiation-induced sarcomas have a poor sarcoma-related survival? Br J Cancer 2012;106(2):297–306.

47. de Jong MA, Oldenborg S, Bing Oei S, et al. Reirradiation and hyperthermia for radiation-associated sarcoma. Cancer 2012;118(1):180–7.

48. Lagrange JL, Ramaioli A, Chateau MC, et al. Sarcoma after radiation therapy: retrospective multiinstitutional study of 80 histologically confirmed cases. Radiation Therapist and Pathologist Groups of the Federation Nationale des Centres de Lutte Contre le Cancer. Radiology 2000;216(1):197–205.

Primary Tumors of the Osseous Chest Wall and Their Management

Mathew Thomas, MD[a],*, K Robert Shen, MD[b]

KEYWORDS

• Chest wall tumors • Bone tumors • Chest wall resection and reconstruction • Fibrous dysplasia

KEY POINTS

• Primary osseous chest wall tumors are rare and may be malignant or benign.
• Wide surgical resection provides a high rate of cure in many primary tumors of the chest wall.
• A multidisciplinary team approach should be strongly considered when dealing with these tumors.
• Proper reconstruction of the chest wall after resection of tumors is important in restoring function and stability.

INTRODUCTION

Primary tumors of the chest wall can arise from either the soft tissues or the bony rib cage. The rib cage is an important part of the axial skeleton and is composed of the ribs, costal cartilages, and sternum. The clavicles and scapula are sometimes included in descriptions of the rib cage[1] but they are parts of the shoulder girdle.

Primary chest wall tumors are uncommon and account for less than 2% of all new primary tumors.[2] Secondary tumors are more common and may occur by hematogenous metastases or direct invasion from the lung, mediastinum, pleura, or breast.[3,4] Approximately 55% of primary malignant chest wall tumors originate from bone or cartilage and the remaining 45% from the soft tissues.[5]

Primary tumors of the bony chest wall are rare and account for only 5.9% to 8% of all bone tumors.[6,7] These bone tumors can arise either spontaneously or as part of familial syndromes. Risk factors for developing chest wall tumors include prior trauma or radiation exposure for treatment of other malignancies such as breast cancer or lymphoma.[8,9] Nearly 85% of primary bone tumors originate in the ribs and the remaining 15% in the sternum. Almost all sternal tumors are malignant, compared with about 88% of rib tumors.[10] Although most malignant chest wall tumors occur in adults, when chest wall tumors are seen in children they are almost always malignant.[11,12] Primary chest wall tumors account for 26% to 44% of chest wall resections that were performed at major academic medical centers.[4,13–15]

This article describes the features of the most common primary osseous tumors of the chest wall and their management.

CLASSIFICATION

Primary osseous chest wall tumors are commonly classified as either malignant or benign. The distinction between the various tumors based on their cell of origin or cause is not often clear because many osseous tumors show mixed cellularity, making a precise pathologic diagnosis often challenging.[16] However, tumors have been traditionally classified according to their proposed tissue of origin, as shown in **Table 1**.

[a] Division of Cardiothoracic Surgery, Mayo Clinic, 4500 San Pablo Road, Jacksonville, FL 32224, USA; [b] Division of General Thoracic Surgery, Mayo Clinic, 200 First Street Southwest, Rochester, MN 55905, USA
* Corresponding author.
E-mail address: Thomas.mathew@mayo.edu

Thorac Surg Clin 27 (2017) 181–193
http://dx.doi.org/10.1016/j.thorsurg.2017.01.012
1547-4127/17/© 2017 Elsevier Inc. All rights reserved.

Table 1
Classification of primary osseous chest wall tumors

Primary Tissue of Origin	Benign	Malignant
Bone	Osteoblastoma Osteoid osteoma	Osteosarcoma
Cartilage	Chondroma Osteochondroma Benign chondroblastoma	Chondrosarcoma
Fibrous tissue	Fibrous dysplasia	—
Bone marrow	Eosinophilic granuloma	Solitary plasmacytoma
Osteoclast	Giant cell tumor (osteoclastoma)	—
Vascular	Hemangioma	Hemangiosarcoma
Undetermined	Aneurysmal bone cyst	Ewing sarcoma

CLINICAL PRESENTATION

Most osseous tumors of the chest wall cause pain as the most common symptom, with or without a palpable mass.[5,17] In contrast, most soft tissue tumors present initially as a painless mass.[18] The presenting pain can be chronic and generalized, which causes it to be frequently managed as nonspecific musculoskeletal pain. Occasionally, trauma to the chest directs the attention of the patient to the underlying tumor, which may then be mistaken for a traumatic swelling. In about 20% of patients, an asymptomatic bone tumor is incidentally found on radiographic imaging done for other purposes.[19] In the case of some bone tumors, such as Ewing sarcoma and Langerhans cell histiocytosis, systemic symptoms such as fever, malaise, and generalized nonspecific bone pain may be the presenting symptoms. Because of the wide variations in presentation, it is not possible to differentiate benign and malignant lesions based on symptoms alone.[20]

EVALUATION
History and Physical Examination

Because most patients seeking a surgical opinion for a chest wall tumor have already been found to have a physical or radiographic abnormality, the role of the thoracic surgeon is to diagnose the underlying condition and determine the appropriate management. The presence of any chest wall mass in a child or a sternal mass in an adult should immediately raise the suspicion of a malignant tumor.

Evaluation begins with a detailed history that should include questions about prior malignancies, radiation, or trauma to the chest. A history of prior radiation to the chest not only increases the suspicion of a radiation-induced malignant bone tumor but also affects wound healing and reconstructive options after resection. The

patient's performance status should be properly assessed to determine whether surgical resection could be tolerated. Comorbidities such as chronic obstructive pulmonary disease, smoking, morbid obesity, uncontrolled diabetes mellitus, and other debilitating illnesses may be risk factors for increased complications after surgery.

Physical examination often helps to confirm the presence of an underlying tumor and is very important in surgical planning. The size and location of the tumor on the chest wall should be noted, because this determines how to proceed with further management, including biopsy, resection, and reconstruction. A hard, immobile mass fixed to the underlying chest wall should raise the suspicion of a bone tumor. Posterior subscapular tumors or a small anterior tumor under breast tissue may be difficult to examine properly.

Imaging

Almost all osseous tumors can be seen on conventional chest radiographs but may be missed in the early stages when the tumor is small or confined within the contour of the bone. Many tumors have pathognomonic characteristics seen on radiographs that are often sufficient for diagnosis without the need for pretreatment tissue diagnosis. These classic radiographic features are not necessarily seen on more advanced imaging techniques such as computed tomography (CT) or MRI.

Both CT and MRI scans have a critical role to play in surgical planning because the image resolution provided by these technologies often helps in delineating the extent of the tumor and involvement of nearby structures. Tumors originating from the ribcage and spine are best evaluated with CT scans of the chest, which also allow the lungs and mediastinum to be examined for any evidence of pulmonary or nodal metastases. The authors have found CT with three-dimensional (3D) reconstruction of the chest wall to be a useful tool in evaluating the tumor from multiple angles and in planning the options for resection and reconstruction. For patients with very complex tumors, particularly those involving the superior sulcus, which may have involvement of the brachial plexus and/or vascular structures, the authors have also found making models using advanced 3D printers to be useful in surgical planning (**Fig. 1**). The models provide enhanced understanding and visualization of the relationships of critical structures to one another as well as the tumor and also can be used to practice or simulate surgical procedures used for the resection and reconstruction of the chest wall.

MRI scan with contrast is an invaluable test when involvement of the overlying soft tissue, muscle, or adjacent neurovascular structures is a concern. Vascular structures can be visualized with either MRI or CT using intravascular contrast, but MRI may provide better resolution of the tissue planes between the tumor and the vessel wall. Similarly, posterior chest wall tumors that seem to involve the spine or spinal cord are best assessed with MRI scans.

PET scans and radionucleotide bone scans are more useful in staging and may identify additional foci of tumor in other bones or distant metastases. PET is also highly accurate in determining response to treatment of sarcomas.[21]

Tissue Diagnosis

Although radiographic imaging can identify many types of bone tumors, a tissue biopsy is often used to confirm the diagnosis, to rule out metastatic lesions, or when surgery is not considered as primary treatment. Techniques for obtaining tissue include percutaneous core needle biopsy, incisional biopsy, or excisional biopsy. Core needle biopsy has been shown to have a high accuracy for bone tumors and in some series was reported to be comparable with incisional biopsy.[22,23] The disadvantages of core needle biopsy include the inability to distinguish between certain benign and malignant tumors and the limited amount of tissue available for further testing. Incisional biopsy is preferred for tumors that are larger than 5 cm. The incision should be oriented in such a way that allows resection of the biopsy site when definitive resection is performed later. The most direct route for biopsy should be selected without undermining or raising skin flaps. Excisional biopsy is preferred if tumor is small enough to be resected up front easily with wide margins of at least 2 cm.

BENIGN TUMORS
Osteochondroma (Osteocartilaginous Exostosis)

Clinical features
Osteochondroma is the most common benign osseous tumor of the chest wall, accounting for about 50% of benign rib tumors. It is a cortical tumor that arises from the metaphyseal region of the rib and consists of both bone and cartilage tissue. Men are affected 3 times more often than women, with a predilection for younger ages. It may present as a solitary, long-standing, painless, palpable mass with outward expansion or may remain asymptomatic with inward growth into the bone. Multiple osteochondromas can occur de novo or as part of an autosomal dominant familial condition called hereditary multiple exostoses.

Radiographic finding
The typical radiographic appearance of osteochondroma is a pedunculated or sessile mass

A   **B**

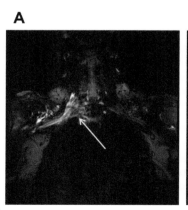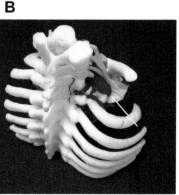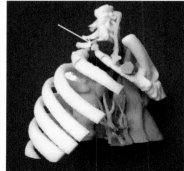

Fig. 1. (*A*) MRI of chest showing Pancoast tumor (*arrow*) of lung invading brachial plexus and first and second ribs. (*B*) Different views of 3D printed model of the chest showing Pancoast tumor (*blue color/arrow*) invading ribs and lower trunk of brachial plexus.

with an overlying cartilage cap, projecting from the surface of the bone via an osseous stalk. A thin, calcified rim is sometimes seen on the cartilage cap. CT or MRI scans are useful in showing the continuity of the lesion with the bone and also in assessing the thickness of the cartilaginous cap. A 2-mm to 3-mm, thin, smooth, regular cap is almost always benign, whereas a cap greater than 2 cm in thickness usually indicates a secondary chondrosarcoma.[24]

Prognosis and management

The risk of malignant degeneration in osteochondromas is unknown but is considered to be probably less than 1%; malignancy may be indicated by extensive calcification and radiolucent irregularities of the cartilage cap.[25]

Resection of osteochondroma is not generally indicated in asymptomatic prepubescent patients except in cases of enlarging tumors or when uncharacteristic radiographic findings are present. When detected past puberty, osteochondromas should be completely resected because of the risks of pathologic fractures and malignant transformation. The best technique to ensure complete resection is to remove the lesion en bloc as a segment of the rib with grossly negative margins.[24] Recurrence may occur if the cartilaginous cap is not completely resected and was reported in slightly more than 2% of all osteochondromas seen at the Mayo Clinic.[24]

Chondromas (Enchondromas)

Clinical features

Chondromas are benign cartilaginous tumors that arise from the costochondral junction of the chest wall, representing about 15% of all benign rib tumors. Although almost all chondroid neoplasms of the sternum are malignant, the occasional benign sternal tumor is most often a chondroma.[26] Grossly, the tumor is composed of confluent masses of bluish, semitranslucent hyaline cartilage with a distinctly lobular arrangement. They affect both sexes equally and present typically between the second and third decades of life as slowly enlarging, painless masses along the anterior aspect of the chest wall.

Radiographic features

Chondroma appears as a slow-growing, expansile, osteolytic mass arising from the medulla of the bone with a thin cortical shell. There may be matrix mineralization consisting of punctate calcifications and endosteal scalloping of the cortex may be evident.[27] MRI may reveal the classic appearance of hyaline cartilage within a lobulated mass when calcifications are not present on CT or radiographs.

Prognosis and management

The clinical and radiographic features of chondromas and chondrosarcomas overlap significantly. Even histologic differentiation between chondromas and low-grade chondrosarcomas can be difficult. For this reason, all chondromas should be considered malignant and managed surgically with wide local resection.[10] Core needle or incisional biopsies are not recommended because they do not rule out a malignant component. Although society guidelines for surveillance for recurrence of chondromas do not currently exist, serial imaging to detect local recurrence should be considered if chondrosarcoma has not been completely ruled out on surgical pathology. MRI may be preferred to CT for monitoring purposes to avoid radiation exposure in patients with chondroma, who are often young.

Fibrous Dysplasia

Clinical features

Fibrous dysplasia is a neoplastic condition in which the medulla of the rib is gradually replaced by fibrous tissue. This process produces an expansile and cystic mass along the lateral or posterolateral aspect of the rib. Although usually asymptomatic, fibrous dysplasia may present with localized rib pain, as a solitary tender mass, or with pathologic fractures. It may also be discovered incidentally when chest radiographs or scans are done for other reasons.

In McCune-Albright syndrome, fibrous dysplasia may occur in multiple bones throughout the body, causing multiple pathologic fractures and severe bone pain. Other features of this syndrome include yellow or brown skin pigmentation (café-au-lait spots) and multiple endocrine hyperfunction causing precocious puberty in girls.

Radiographic features

Fibrous dysplasia appears on radiographs as well-defined zones of rarefaction. A cystic or intramedullary trabeculated lesion (ground-glass appearance) along the posterior aspect of the rib may be seen in long-standing lesions. With continued growth, the tumor expands outward, leading to a thin rim of sclerotic cortex.

Prognosis and management

In asymptomatic patients, especially children, conservative management is sufficient because the lesions may stop growing when puberty is reached. Surgical resection may be indicated in patients with pain or fracture, or to rule out malignancy. Malignant degeneration seems to be generally associated with a prior history of radiation treatment of fibrous dysplasia.[28] Spontaneous malignant degeneration into sarcoma without prior history of radiation is rare but has also been reported.[28–30]

Long-term bisphosphonates have been used in McCune-Albright syndrome with some success[31] but no evidence currently exists for their use in isolated fibrous dysplasia of the ribs.

Langerhans Cell Histiocytosis (Eosinophilic Granuloma, Histiocytosis X)

Clinical features
Langerhans cell histiocytosis (LCH) is the localized manifestation of a group of 3 conditions that are characterized by the pathognomonic histologic finding of foci of proliferating histiocytes. The other two conditions are Schuller-Christian disease and Letterer-Siwe disease, which are more disseminated and aggressive forms.

Patients with bone lesions caused by LCH present with a solitary, painful area that is usually associated with a palpable or visible mass in the chest. In addition to pain, systemic symptoms such as fevers and malaise may also be presenting features and can indicate a more disseminated form of the disease. Pulmonary involvement is seen in some patients as diffuse lung lesions and sometimes causes spontaneous pneumothorax.

Radiographic features
On radiography, LCH appears as discrete, lytic, and expansile lesions in the bone that destroy the cortex. Thick and solid subperiosteal new bone formation is also seen. In flat bones such as the clavicle, the lesion may be poorly defined with erosion of the cortex and may be diagnosed as a malignant lesion.[32]

Prognosis and management
In the case of single lesion of LCH, observation in asymptomatic patients is sufficient. Spontaneous regression may occur and has been reported after smoking cessation.[33] If symptomatic, local radiation or excision of the lesion may be considered. When multiple lesions are present, there is hardly any role for surgery and systemic therapy with chemotherapy or corticosteroids is usually the treatment of choice.

Aneurysmal Bone Cyst

Clinical features
These are neoplastic bone cysts of unknown pathogenesis. They have been known to occur after a fracture or de novo without a precedent lesion and thus may be a reactive response leading to neoplastic changes.[34] They present before the age of 20 years in 75% of cases. Patients mostly complain of pain and swelling associated with a palpable mass or pathologic fractures. Differential diagnoses of aneurysmal bone cysts include osteosarcoma and giant cell tumor. Telangiectatic osteosarcoma can be especially difficult to distinguish from an aneurysmal bone cyst by radiography or gross pathology alone. However, the histologic presence of pleomorphic-appearing cells in the septa is characteristic of telangiectatic osteosarcoma.

Radiographic features
Aneurysmal bone cyst appears as a lucent, eccentric lesion in the medullary cavity, with a thin rim of calcification and internal septations (**Fig. 2**). The septations, which may contain hemorrhagic fluid levels, are best seen on CT or MRI scans. Occasionally, a solid aneurysmal bone cyst without any cystic spaces or septations is seen.

Prognosis and management
Resection with grossly negative margins is recommended for symptomatic bone cysts or if malignancy is suspected. Aneurysmal bone cysts have been reported to spontaneously regress even when incompletely resected or after incisional biopsy. Occasional malignant transformation of

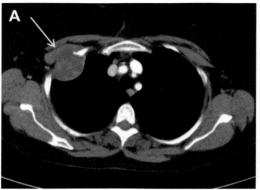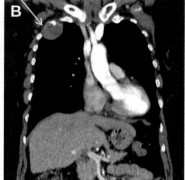

Fig. 2. (A, B) CT views of second rib aneurysmal bone cyst (*arrow*) showing internal septations.

these benign tumors into sarcoma has been reported after radiation therapy and curettage.

MALIGNANT TUMORS
Chondrosarcoma

Clinical features
Chondrosarcoma is the most common primary osseous tumor of the chest wall[4] and resembles chondroma both clinically and radiographically. It arises anteriorly at the costochondral junction or sternum and consists of cartilaginous tissue (**Fig. 3**). A history of crushing injury to the chest wall was present in 12.5% of patients who were treated for chondrosarcoma at our institution, suggesting an association with trauma.[9]

Chondrosarcoma usually presents between the third and fifth decades as a slowly growing, initially painless mass that can become painful with time. It affects men more often than women. This tumor is typically not very aggressive and has a low risk of early metastasis.

Radiographic features
The radiographic features of chondrosarcomas, especially when low grade, and chondromas are too similar to be able to distinguish one entity from the other.

Prognosis and management
Wide surgical resection of all anterior costal cartilaginous tumors should be performed because it is difficult to distinguish a benign chondroma from a malignant chondrosarcoma. Chondrosarcomas do not respond to chemotherapy or radiation therapy but have been shown in our institutional series to have 10-year survival of up to 96% when wide resection is performed, compared with 65% for local excision.[9] Overall survival rates of patients with chondrosarcoma in major cancer institutions have been reported to range from 64% at 5 years to 53% at 10 years.[9,17]

Osteosarcoma

Clinical features
This is a rare but very aggressive tumor that has a bimodal age distribution, occurring initially in the second and third decades and then after the sixth decade of life. It has a slight preponderance in men. Postradiation osteosarcoma of the ribs occurs in older patients and has a higher incidence in women. Osteosarcoma presents as a painful mass because of rapid enlargement. Clinically, it may be difficult to determine whether the overlying soft tissues are involved because the tumor tends to grow outward into the soft tissues. Increased serum alkaline phosphatase level caused by osteoblastic activity is seen in about 50% of the patients. Patients with osteosarcomas may have synchronous metastases at their initial presentation or develop distant metastases later.[35]

Radiographic findings
The pathognomonic radiograph finding in osteosarcoma is the sunburst appearance, with rays of calcification radiating outward from the cortex of the bone. There is significant bone destruction with effacement of the borders between normal and involved bone. CT and MRI can help to delineate the extent of disease, including the involvement of other bones in multicentric osteosarcoma.

Treatment and prognosis
The prognosis of osteosarcomas has historically been very poor even with adjuvant chemotherapy because of early distant metastases.[5] Encouragingly, significant changes in management of osteosarcoma have improved overall survival over the past few decades. A 5-year survival rate of up to 78% was reported after chemotherapy, surgical resection, and postoperative radiation in a retrospective study that included 9 patients with osteosarcoma of the chest wall.[36] Staging at the time of

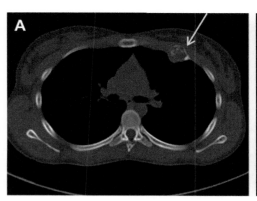
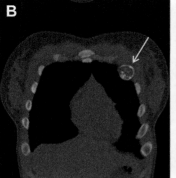
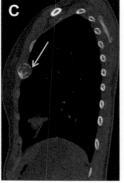

Fig. 3. (A–C) CT views of low-grade chondrosarcoma (*arrow*) of the third rib.

diagnosis is important to determine the appropriate treatment. Pulmonary metastases should be ruled out with CT scans of the chest. Induction chemotherapy with wide local resection is the standard treatment and has significantly improved outcomes.

Ewing Sarcoma

Clinical features

Ewing sarcoma is not a single type of tumor but a family of very aggressive and rapidly growing, small, basophilic (blue), round to oval cell, primary osseous tumors that share many histologic and immunohistochemical features. Because of similarities in immunohistochemical, cytogenetic, and molecular features between primitive neuroectodermal tumors (PNETs) and Ewing sarcoma, they are now considered to be a single Ewing sarcoma family originating from neuroectodermal cells, in various stages of differentiation.[37]

Occasionally, Ewing sarcoma originates in extraskeletal tissues. Osseous Ewing sarcoma is rare in adults but is the most common primary chest wall tumor in children, especially boys. Three-quarters of patients are affected in the first 2 decades of life.[37] The tumor can metastasize to the lungs, lymph nodes, and other long bones.

Clinical features of Ewing sarcoma include systemic symptoms such as fever, malaise, and loss of weight along with a painful, tender rib mass. Laboratory findings include leukocytosis, anemia, and increased erythrocyte sedimentation rate. Presentation with systemic features is associated with worse prognosis. Ewing sarcoma can be difficult to distinguish from other tumors that have round cells.

One variety of PNET of the chest wall is called Askin tumor. This tumor presents as an extremely large mass with severe bone destruction but also tends to grow inward to involve the underlying lung[38] (Fig. 4).

Radiographic findings

The characteristic radiograph finding of Ewing sarcoma is the presence of onionskin appearance on the surface of the bone caused by the multiple layers of subperiosteal reactive new bone formation. However, the radiographic appearance in advanced Ewing sarcoma may be nonspecific and can overlap with a wide variety of other bone neoplasms and osteomyelitis caused by the destruction of bone along with activation of osteoblasts. With severe destruction of the cortex, the tumor may merge into the surrounding soft tissues. This condition may be seen as subtle channels that extend through the cortex at CT or MR imaging or as radiating spicules on radiographs.

Prognosis and management

Ewing sarcomas respond well to multiagent preoperative chemotherapy. With the use of preoperative chemotherapy, the extent of chest wall resection required is less and there is a greater chance of obtaining complete resection. Significant improvement in survival has been reported with chemotherapy followed by complete resection.[39] According to the European Intergroup Ewing Sarcoma Study group, rib involvement had a good prognosis compared with other areas in the body.[40] Postoperative radiation has a role in the local control of Ewing sarcoma that has not been completely resected but does not seem to improve survival for completely resected tumors.[41]

GENERAL PRINCIPLES OF MANAGEMENT

There is a wide variety of both benign and malignant bone tumors and the decision regarding management is made based on diagnosis, site, and size of the individual tumor. In the case of malignant tumors, the stage at the time of presentation is also important in determining the appropriate treatment. Other considerations include

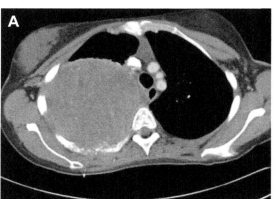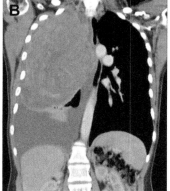

Fig. 4. (A, B) CT of the chest showing giant Ewing tumor (Askin variety) of the fourth rib extending into the chest.

the age of the patient and presence of other comorbidities. A multidisciplinary team approach that involves thoracic surgeons, medical and radiation oncologists, and plastic surgeons should be used to enable the best possible outcomes for patients with chest wall tumors.

Surgical Management

In general, wide local resection is the primary treatment of most bone tumors localized to the chest wall. Chemotherapy and radiation therapy in the neoadjuvant or adjuvant setting may also be included with surgery as part of multimodality therapy. Certain tumors, such as LCH and solitary plasmacytomas, are treated medically with chemotherapy, corticosteroids, or radiation, and do not usually require surgical resection.

The chest wall plays an important role in respiratory physiology and dynamics. It also protects the thoracic and upper abdominal organs from injury. Surgical resection of a portion of the chest wall can adversely affect these functions and may also create significant cosmetic defects. Hence, surgical management of chest wall tumors requires not just an understanding about the principles of resection but also a sound knowledge regarding reconstruction of the chest wall. Fear of reconstructing the chest wall should not limit the extent of resection necessary to prevent recurrence. If an extensive resection and reconstruction is beyond the expertise of the surgeon, the patient should be referred to an institution with significant experience in dealing with chest wall tumors. Once the tissue planes have been violated, the chance for achieving adequate local control diminishes even with subsequent wider resection. Inadequately resected chest wall sarcomas have a high recurrence rate of 86%, which can be even higher at 96% when subsequent nonradical resection is performed for recurrent tumors.[42]

The recommended extent of resection depends on the type of tumor and its degree of aggressiveness. A resection margin of 4 cm was shown to nearly double (56% vs 29%) the 5-year survival in malignant chest wall tumors compared with a margin of 2 cm in a study of patients treated at the Mayo Clinic.[43] A margin of 2 cm may be sufficient for benign tumors and metastases but not for primary malignant tumors.[10] In order to achieve radical resection, removal of the entire bone, such as sternum or rib, is generally recommended for high-grade neoplasms because of the risk of subperiosteal or intramedullary spread. Radical resection should also include en bloc resection of previous biopsy incision scars and tracks along with the overlying soft tissues, as well as any attached underlying structures, such as pleura, lung, diaphragm, or anterior mediastinal tissues. Recurrent chest wall sarcomas have been shown to require much wider resections and have worse overall and disease-free survival compared with primary chest wall sarcomas.[42]

The use of minimally invasive techniques for resection of chest wall tumors, such as video-assisted thoracic surgery (VATS), and hybrid approaches using open techniques and VATS have been reported.[44–46] These techniques require significant skills in minimally invasive thoracic surgery and preoperative planning. It should be pointed out that long-term oncologic outcomes after minimally invasive resection of chest wall tumors have not been reported to date. In our opinion, until such results are available, minimally invasive surgery should be reserved only for those tumors that have been clearly diagnosed as benign, and only if the procedure can be performed without compromising the principles of oncologic resection.

Reconstruction

Resection of chest wall tumors leaves behind a defect that may need reconstruction to restore function and stability, and to offer protection to the underlying organs. However, not all chest wall defects need repair. In general, defects larger than 5 cm in greatest dimension require some kind of reconstruction (**Fig. 5**). In the case of subscapular defects, reconstruction may not be required when less than 10 cm. These numbers are not absolute and are to be used as general guidelines to determine whether reconstruction is indicated or not. For instance, a small posterior defect may require reconstruction if the tip of the scapula gets entrapped in it.

Reconstructing the chest wall after resection requires proper preoperative planning and preparation. Such planning should involve the plastic surgeons when the reconstruction is determined to be complex. All options for rigid and soft tissue coverage should be carefully explored to determine what is most appropriate for the individual patient. Options for reconstruction are generally classified as rigid, semirigid, or nonrigid (**Table 2**). Nonrigid reconstruction is generally with autologous soft tissue. Rigid and semirigid reconstruction involve the use of prosthetic materials with or without autologous or cadaveric rib grafts. In a series of 500 patients who underwent chest wall reconstruction at our institution, only 37% of patients required prosthetic reconstruction with semirigid material such as polypropylene or polytetrafluoroethylene (PTFE) mesh, or autologous rib reconstruction.[4] In the remaining patients,

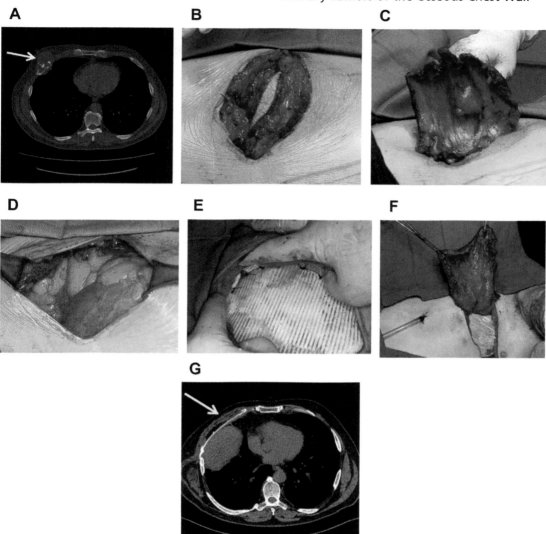

Fig. 5. (*A*) CT view showing chondrosarcoma (*arrow*) of the anterior chest wall. (*B–D*) Intraoperative views showing radical resection of tumor with skin, soft tissues, and ribs. (*E, F*) Intraoperative views showing reconstruction of the resulting defect with polytetrafluoroethylene (PTFE) mesh and latissimus dorsi pedicled flap. (*G*) CT view 6 months after surgery showing PTFE mesh with overlying latissimus dorsi muscle flap (*arrow*).

Table 2
Reconstruction options after chest wall resection

Nonrigid	Rigid	Semirigid

1. Pedicled musculocutaneous flaps
  a. Latissimus dorsi
  b. Transverse rectus abdominis
  c. External oblique
	Methyl methacrylate–polypropylene mesh sandwich	Polypropylene mesh

2. Pedicled flaps
  a. Pectoralis major
  b. Serratus
  c. Omentum
	Rib and sternal metallic plating systems	Polytetrafluoroethylene mesh

3. Free soft tissue flaps	—	—

reconstruction was performed with soft tissue flaps only. Since the publication of that report in 1996, significant advances in reconstructive materials for the chest wall have been made. At present, in addition to the previously mentioned semirigid patches, metallic rib and sternal plating systems are readily available and can span large gaps in the chest wall, adding stability to support (**Fig. 6**).

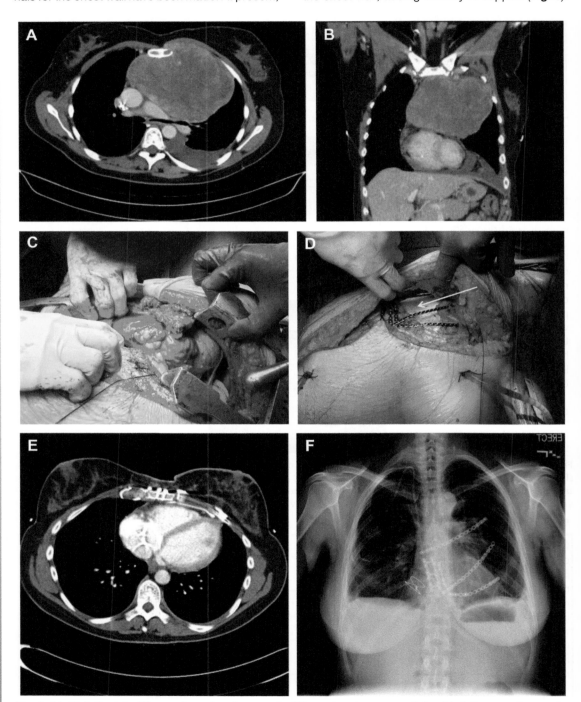

Fig. 6. (*A, B*) Patient A: CT scan views showing poorly differentiated sarcoma of the third rib extending to the sternum and displacing the mediastinal structures. (*C*) Clamshell thoracotomy for resection of large sarcoma in patient A. (*D*) Reconstructed chest wall with underlay PTFE mesh (*arrow*), bridging rib and sternal plates. (*E, F*) Patient A: CT scan and chest radiograph 3 months after resection and reconstruction.

With the increasing availability of 3D printing technology, custom-made prostheses can now be created, expanding the options for reconstruction.[47,48] However, the technology remains expensive and there is a significant amount of time needed to manufacture the prosthesis, which potentially limits more widespread use.

Soft tissue coverage of the defects includes pedicled or free flaps and omentum, and are covered in a separate article in this journal.

Radiation Therapy

The role of radiation therapy in the treatment of localized, completely resectable primary osseous tumors of the chest wall is not well defined. Not all tumors are radiosensitive, and some tumors, such as chondrosarcomas, are not chemosensitive or radiosensitive. Adjuvant radiotherapy is advocated for local control of any remaining tumor cells after surgery. Some studies have shown survival benefit to adding radiation therapy to surgical resection but included both soft tissue and osseous sarcomas, hence limiting conclusions regarding its value in bone tumors.[49] The rare incidence of chest wall tumors also makes it difficult to provide conclusive evidence regarding the best way to manage them. Long-term effects of radiation therapy for treatment of chest wall sarcomas have not been reported, but radiation has been known to affect healing and can even increase the risk of radiation-induced cancers.

Chemotherapy

Neoadjuvant chemotherapy is standard of care in the treatment of bone tumors such as Ewing sarcoma and osteosarcoma.[50] The role of chemotherapy in other tumors that are surgically resectable is controversial.

COMPLICATIONS AND OUTCOMES

Outcomes after treatment of primary chest wall osseous tumors depend on /several factors, including pathology of the tumor and completeness of resection. Complications after surgical resection can also affect survival. Multiple studies in large series of patients with primary chest wall tumors treated at the Mayo Clinic have shown that excellent outcomes can be obtained when aggressive resection is combined with proper reconstruction of the chest wall.[9,51,52]

Morbidity and mortality after chest wall resection remain concerns and are mainly related to the alterations in pulmonary mechanics. Mortalities of up to 7% and morbidity rates of up to 46% have been reported in current large patient series.[53] Respiratory complications are the most common and range from 11% to 24%.[3,51,53] There is no clear evidence that surgical technique or the prosthetic material used can influence the incidence of respiratory complications.[53]

Local infection of the wound and prosthetic material is the other major complication following chest wall resection and reconstruction and is reported to be as high as 20%.[3,53] Slightly more than half of all patients who develop wound infection eventually require removal of the prosthesis.[3,51] Complications following reconstruction with methyl methacrylate Marlex mesh seem to be much more common than after semirigid prosthetic reconstruction using PTFE or polypropylene mesh.[3]

SUMMARY

Primary bone tumors of the chest wall are rare but occur in several pathologic varieties that may be either malignant or benign. Early diagnosis and aggressive surgical resection of most primary chest wall tumors result in excellent long-term outcomes, including cure. Although diagnosis can often be made based on radiologic appearance in bone tumors, some tumors require biopsy for diagnosis. Proper management of any chest wall tumor requires a sound knowledge of the principles of both oncologic resection and chest wall reconstruction. A multidisciplinary team approach is invaluable in management of chest wall tumors and reconstruction of chest wall defects.

REFERENCES

1. Smith SE, Keshavjee S. Primary chest wall tumors. Thorac Surg Clin 2010;20(4):495–507.
2. Perry RR, Venzon D, Roth JA, et al. Survival after surgical resection for high-grade chest wall sarcomas. Ann Thorac Surg 1990;49(3):363–8 [discussion: 368–9].
3. Weyant MJ, Bains MS, Venkatraman E, et al. Results of chest wall resection and reconstruction with and without rigid prosthesis. Ann Thorac Surg 2006; 81(1):279–85.
4. Arnold PG, Pairolero PC. Chest-wall reconstruction: an account of 500 consecutive patients. Plast Reconstr Surg 1996;98(5):804–10.
5. Burt M. Primary malignant tumors of the chest wall. The Memorial Sloan-Kettering Cancer Center experience. Chest Surg Clin N Am 1994;4(1):137–54.
6. Teitelbaum SL. Twenty years' experience with intrinsic tumors of the bony thorax at a large institution. J Thorac Cardiovasc Surg 1972;63(5):776–82.
7. Unni KK, Inwards CY. Introduction and scope of study. In: Unni KK, Inwards CY, editors. Dahlin's

bone tumors. 6th edition. Philadelphia: Wolters Kluwer; 2009. p. 1–8.

8. Schwarz RE, Burt M. Radiation-associated malignant tumors of the chest wall. Ann Surg Oncol 1996;3(4):387–92.

9. McAfee MK, Pairolero PC, Bergstralh EJ, et al. Chondrosarcoma of the chest wall: factors affecting survival. Ann Thorac Surg 1985;40(6):535–41.

10. Allen MS. Chest wall tumors. In: Selke FW, del Nido PJ, Swanson SJ, editors. Sabiston & Spencer surgery of the chest, vol. 1. Philadelphia: Saunders Elsevier; 2010. p. 380–7.

11. La Quaglia MP. Chest wall tumors in childhood and adolescence. Semin Pediatr Surg 2008;17(3):173–80.

12. van den Berg H, van Rijn RR, Merks JH. Management of tumors of the chest wall in childhood: a review. J Pediatr Hematol Oncol 2008;30(3):214–21.

13. Martini N, Huvos AG, Burt ME, et al. Predictors of survival in malignant tumors of the sternum. J Thorac Cardiovasc Surg 1996;111(1):96–105 [discussion: 105–6].

14. Mansour KA, Thourani VH, Losken A, et al. Chest wall resections and reconstruction: a 25-year experience. Ann Thorac Surg 2002;73(6):1720–5 [discussion: 1725–6.

15. Hsu PK, Hsu HS, Lee HC, et al. Management of primary chest wall tumors: 14 years' clinical experience. J Chin Med Assoc 2006;69(8):377–82.

16. Faber LP, Somers J, Templeton AC. Chest wall tumors. Curr Probl Surg 1995;32(8):661–747.

17. Burt M, Fulton M, Wessner-Dunlap S, et al. Primary bony and cartilaginous sarcomas of chest wall: results of therapy. Ann Thorac Surg 1992;54(2):226–32.

18. Gordon MS, Hajdu SI, Bains MS, et al. Soft tissue sarcomas of the chest wall. Results of surgical resection. J Thorac Cardiovasc Surg 1991;101(5):843–54.

19. Sabanathan S, Salama FD, Morgan WE, et al. Primary chest wall tumors. Ann Thorac Surg 1985;39(1):4–15.

20. Athanassiadi K, Kalavrouziotis G, Rondogianni D, et al. Primary chest wall tumors: early and long-term results of surgical treatment. Eur J Cardiothorac Surg 2001;19(5):589–93.

21. Piperkova E, Mikhaeil M, Mousavi A, et al. Impact of PET and CT in PET/CT studies for staging and evaluating treatment response in bone and soft tissue sarcomas. Clin Nucl Med 2009;34(3):146–50.

22. Kiatisevi P, Thanakit V, Sukunthanak B, et al. Computed tomography-guided core needle biopsy versus incisional biopsy in diagnosing musculoskeletal lesions. J Orthop Surg (Hong Kong) 2013;21(2):204–8.

23. Trieu J, Schlicht SM, Choong PF. Diagnosing musculoskeletal tumours: how accurate is CT-guided core needle biopsy? Eur J Surg Oncol 2016;42(7):1049–56.

24. Unni KK, Inwards CY. Chondrosarcoma (primary, secondary, dedifferentiated, and clear cell). In: Unni KK, Inwards CY, editors. Dahlin's bone tumors. 6th edition. Philadelphia: Wolter Kluwer; 2009. p. 60–91.

25. Peterson HA. Multiple hereditary osteochondromata. Clin Orthop Relat Res 1989;(239):222–30.

26. Unni KK, Inwards CY. Chondroma. In: Unni KK, Inwards CY, editors. Dahlin's bone tumors. 6th edition. Philadelphia: Wolter Kluwer; 2009. p. 22–40.

27. Hughes EK, James SL, Butt S, et al. Benign primary tumours of the ribs. Clin Radiol 2006;61(4):314–22.

28. Ruggieri P, Sim FH, Bond JR, et al. Malignancies in fibrous dysplasia. Cancer 1994;73(5):1411–24.

29. Reis C, Genden EM, Bederson JB, et al. A rare spontaneous osteosarcoma of the calvarium in a patient with long-standing fibrous dysplasia: CT and MR findings. Br J Radiol 2008;81(962):e31–4.

30. Van Rossem C, Pauwels P, Somville J, et al. Sarcomatous degeneration in fibrous dysplasia of the rib cage. Ann Thorac Surg 2013;96(4):e89–90.

31. Lala R, Matarazzo P, Andreo M, et al. Bisphosphonate treatment of bone fibrous dysplasia in McCune-Albright syndrome. J Pediatr Endocrinol Metab 2006;19(Suppl 2):583–93.

32. Unni KK, Inwards CY. Conditions that commonly simulate primary neoplasms of bone. In: Unni KK, Inwards CY, editors. Dahlin's bone tumors. 6th edition. Philadelphia: Wolter Kluwer; 2009. p. 305–80.

33. Routy B, Hoang J, Gruber J. Pulmonary Langerhans cell histiocytosis with lytic bone involvement in an adult smoker: regression following smoking cessation. Case Rep Hematol 2015;2015:201536.

34. Cottalorda J, Bourelle S. Modern concepts of primary aneurysmal bone cyst. Arch Orthop Trauma Surg 2007;127(2):105–14.

35. Park BJ, Flores RM. Chest wall tumors. In: Shields TW, LoCicero J, Reed CE, et al, editors. General thoracic surgery, vol. 1, 7th edition. Philadelphia: Lippincott Williams & Wilkins; 2005. p. 669–77.

36. Lin GQ, Li YQ, Huang LJ, et al. Chest wall tumors: diagnosis, treatment and reconstruction. Exp Ther Med 2015;9(5):1807–12.

37. Unni KK, Inwards CY. Ewing tumor. In: Unni KK, Inwards CY, editors. Dahlin's bone tumor. 6th edition. Philadelphia: Wolter Kluwer; 2009. p. 211–24.

38. Winer-Muram HT, Kauffman WM, Gronemeyer SA, et al. Primitive neuroectodermal tumors of the chest wall (Askin tumors): CT and MR findings. AJR Am J Roentgenol 1993;161(2):265–8.

39. Krasin MJ, Davidoff AM, Rodriguez-Galindo C, et al. Definitive surgery and multiagent systemic therapy for patients with localized Ewing sarcoma family of

tumors: local outcome and prognostic factors. Cancer 2005;104(2):367–73.

40. Cotterill SJ, Ahrens S, Paulussen M, et al. Prognostic factors in Ewing's tumor of bone: analysis of 975 patients from the European Intergroup Cooperative Ewing's Sarcoma Study Group. J Clin Oncol 2000; 18(17):3108–14.

41. Bedetti B, Wiebe K, Ranft A, et al. Local control in Ewing sarcoma of the chest wall: results of the EURO-EWING 99 trial. Ann Surg Oncol 2015;22(9): 2853–9.

42. Wouters MW, van Geel AN, Nieuwenhuis L, et al. Outcome after surgical resections of recurrent chest wall sarcomas. J Clin Oncol 2008;26(31):5113–8.

43. King RM, Pairolero PC, Trastek VF, et al. Primary chest wall tumors: factors affecting survival. Ann Thorac Surg 1986;41(6):597–601.

44. Gera PK, La Hei E, Cummins G, et al. Thoracoscopy in chest wall Ewing's sarcoma. J Laparoendosc Adv Surg Tech A 2006;16(5):509–12.

45. Abicht TO, de Hoyos AL. Chest wall resection and reconstruction: a true thoracoscopic approach. Innovations (Phila) 2011;6(6):399–402.

46. Hennon MW, Demmy TL. Thoracoscopic resection and re-resection of an anterior chest wall chondrosarcoma. Innovations (Phila) 2012;7(6):445–7.

47. Aragon J, Perez Mendez I. Dynamic 3D printed titanium copy prosthesis: a novel design for large chest wall resection and reconstruction. J Thorac Dis 2016;8(6):E385–9.

48. Aranda JL, Jimenez MF, Rodriguez M, et al. Tridimensional titanium-printed custom-made prosthesis for sternocostal reconstruction. Eur J Cardiothorac Surg 2015;48(4):e92–4.

49. Burt A, Berriochoa J, Korpak A, et al. Treatment of chest wall sarcomas: a single-institution experience over 20 years. Am J Clin Oncol 2015; 38(1):80–6.

50. Girelli L, Luksch R, Podda MG, et al. Surgical approach to primary tumors of the chest wall in children and adolescents: 30 years of mono-institutional experience. Tumori 2016;102(1):89–95.

51. Deschamps C, Tirnaksiz BM, Darbandi R, et al. Early and long-term results of prosthetic chest wall reconstruction. J Thorac Cardiovasc Surg 1999;117(3): 588–91 [discussion: 591–2].

52. Pairolero PC, Arnold PG. Chest wall tumors. Experience with 100 consecutive patients. J Thorac Cardiovasc Surg 1985;90(3):367–72.

53. Hazel K, Weyant MJ. Chest wall resection and reconstruction: management of complications. Thorac Surg Clin 2015;25(4):517–21.

Surgical Management of Lung Cancer Involving the Chest Wall

Michael Lanuti, MD

KEYWORDS

- Lung cancer • Chest wall invasion • En bloc resection

KEY POINTS

- Survival of patients with lung cancer invading the chest wall is highly dependent on completeness of en bloc resection and lymph node involvement.
- Pathologic invasive mediastinal staging will directly influence the ultimate treatment strategy.
- Induction radiation or chemoradiotherapy for lung cancers invading the chest wall outside of the superior sulcus is poorly defined.
- When performing chest wall resection, a 1 cm margin in all directions is generally accepted.
- Chest wall defects less than 5 cm can be managed without reconstruction.

INTRODUCTION

The prevalence of chest wall invasion by nonsmall cell lung cancer is less than 10% in published surgical series. These tumors are given a T3 or T4 designation in the seventh edition TNM staging depending on chest wall or vertebral body invasion.[1] The T designation for invasion of chest wall or vertebral body will remain unchanged in the eighth edition TNM staging.[2] Long-term survival in patients harboring this locally aggressive neoplasm has been associated with complete (R0) resection and node-negative disease.[3–5] Preoperative radiation and en bloc resection were promulgated in the 1950s by Shaw and Paulson for tumors in the thoracic inlet.[6] This strategy remained the standard of care until the 1990s, when neoadjuvant chemotherapy and radiation were investigated. Since that time, induction therapy strategies have been primarily elucidated in Pancoast tumors,[7–9] where efficacy in chest wall invasion outside of the superior sulcus is poorly defined.

The first demonstration of a successful chest wall resection in continuity with a lung cancer was published in 1947 by Coleman, where (3/4) patients undergoing pneumonectomy experienced freedom from disease at 5 months to 6 years after the operation.[10] In subsequent decades, there have been retrospective series from single institutions that have attempted to address prognostic factors.[8,11–14] Advances in the technical approach to removing superior sulcus tumors were described by Dartevelle and colleagues in 1993.[15] The field appeared to move forward again in the prospective evaluation of patients with Pancoast tumors when results of a multi-institutional phase II trial (Southwest Oncology Group 9416) was published in 2007.[16] This study involved 76 surgeons from all North American cooperative groups to enroll 110 patients with T3-4 disease who received 2 cycles of cisplatin and etoposide concurrently with 45 Gy radiation. This cohort achieved 54% 5-year survival after complete resection. Pathologic complete response or minimal microscopic disease was identified in 56%

Disclosure Statement: No commercial or financial conflicts. There are no funding sources.
Division of Thoracic Surgery, Massachusetts General Hospital, Harvard Medical School, 55 Fruit Street, Founders 7, Boston, MA 02114, USA
E-mail address: MLanuti@mgh.harvard.edu

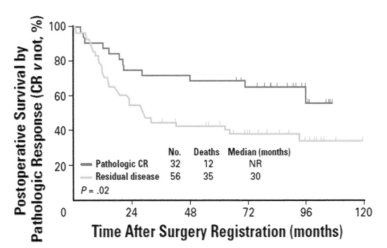

Fig. 1. Results of SWOG 9416 comparing overall survival in patients who achieved a complete pathologic response (CR) versus residual disease. (*From* Rusch VW, Giroux DJ, Kraut MJ, et al. Induction chemoradiation and surgical resection for superior sulcus non-small-cell lung carcinomas: long-term results of Southwest Oncology Group Trial 9416 (Intergroup Trial 0160). J Clin Oncol 2007;25(3):316; with permission.)

of resected specimens (**Fig. 1**). This was corroborated in a phase II Japanese Clinical Oncology Group Trial 9806 where patients were treated with induction chemoradiotherapy (56%, 5-year overall survival) followed by en bloc resection.[17] Employing this paradigm to lung cancers invading the chest wall outside of the superior sulcus has not been well studied.

CLINICAL PRESENTATION

The most common clinical presentation of chest wall invasion in patients diagnosed with primary bronchogenic carcinoma is pain. Although localized chest pain is a strong indication of chest wall involvement, the absence of pain does not exclude the possibility. In 1 study, 7.5% of patients with tumor extending to the periosteum did not have pain.[18] Another important aspect in the early management of a lung tumor involving the chest wall is histologic confirmation of the disease. Differentiating lung cancer from a primary tumor of the chest wall extending into lung will greatly influence the treatment plan. Given the complexity of these locally aggressive neoplasms, patients should routinely be evaluated by a multidisciplinary team including neurosurgery, orthopedic spine surgery, and/or plastic surgery when appropriate.

PRINCIPLES OF SURGICAL TREATMENT

Similar to any patient diagnosed with lung cancer, adequate staging is paramount, particularly in patients harboring lung cancer invading or abutting any part of the chest wall. Patients should undergo diagnostic quality computed tomography (CT) of the chest, positron emission tomography (PET) with attenuation correction CT and brain MRI to rule out intracranial disease given the more

aggressive phenotype of these tumors. Chest or spine MRI can be obtained to delineate encroachment of tumor into the vertebral foramen, or brachial plexus and subclavian vessels in the case of superior sulcus tumors. MRI with respiratory gating has a distinct advantage of demonstrating independent movements of the lung and chest wall, therefore improving the sensitivity of tumor invasion into parietal pleura or diaphragm.[19] If complete en bloc resection is achievable, MRI will not necessarily change the surgical management of tumors located outside of the superior sulcus. If spinal elements are involved, consultation with a spine surgeon will be necessary in planning en bloc resection. Flexible bronchoscopy should not be overlooked, since a subgroup of these patients will present with endobronchial disease that may influence the operative strategy.

Pathologic mediastinal nodal staging is critical to improve patient selection for curative multimodality therapy. This can be achieved by endobronchial ultrasound, cervical mediastinoscopy, anterior mediastinotomy, or video-assisted thoracoscopy. The presence of N2 disease has been reproducibly associated with worse outcome in patients harboring lung cancer with chest wall invasion. Cardillo and colleagues reported an 18% 5-year overall survival for T3N2 disease compared with 61% for T3N0 in 104 patients treated with en bloc resection of lung neoplasms involving the chest wall.[18] In a series of 201 patients treated with en bloc resection, Magdeleinat and colleagues[5] reported 21% 5-year survival in patients with T3N2 disease. No survival difference was noted between patients with N1 or N2 disease. If en bloc resection is being considered, adequate cardiopulmonary reserve must be confirmed by pulmonary function tests and assessment of cardiac function. When performing chest wall resection, a 1 cm margin in all directions is generally accepted; however, some would advocate for obtaining a margin of 1 intact rib above and below the tumor with a 3 to 4 cm lateral margin.[18] Factors that influence the surgical approach to lung cancer invading the chest wall include body habitus, tumor location, and a history of previous radiation. Reconstruction with prosthetic material is predicated on size and site of the chest wall defect. Anterior chest wall defects are often reconstructed with rigid fixation given the proximity of the heart and vital structures. In general, chest wall defects <5 cm can be managed without reconstruction. Posterior chest wall defects under the scapula do not routinely require reconstruction unless the geometry will cause scapular tip entrapment.

Some area of controversy surrounds extrapleural dissection versus en bloc chest wall resection when tumor invades the parietal pleura. This really depends on the presence of bone invasion. The assessment of a tumor-free plane is subjective, where many surgeons perform extrapleural dissection until encountering macroscopic invasion. It should be noted that frozen section specimens composed of soft tissue with bone do not routinely help guide the surgeon intraoperatively, since bone specimens need to be decalcified. Thoracic surgeons should proceed with caution and use extrapleural dissection only in the presence of filmy adhesions with a discernible plane between visceral and parietal pleura. Few published series address this issue. Piehler reported a 75% 5-year survival with en bloc resection in contrast to 28% after an extrapleural resection.[3] Albertucci and colleagues[20] reported a 37.5% rate of local recurrence versus 9.5% in patients undergoing extrapleural resection compared with en bloc chest wall resection, respectively.

ROLE OF SURGERY FOLLOWED BY ADJUVANT THERAPY

In the past 20 years, published literature is sparse on the specific role of radiation in patients with lung cancer and chest wall invasion. Although one may extrapolate from the success of concurrent radiation on superior sulcus tumors, the added benefit of radiation in completely resectable tumors remains unclear. One of the few studies that addressed this issue was published in 1982 from the Toronto group reporting outcomes on 35 patients with completely resected lung cancers invading the chest wall.[21] In those patients who received radiation (N = 13, 8 post-operatively), 56% 5-year survival was reported compared with 30% in nonradiated patients. Overall survival in the entire cohort was 38% at 5 years. In contrast,

postoperative radiation was employed in 74% (139/201) of patients in a larger retrospective population treated with en bloc chest wall resection for invasive lung cancer, where there was no apparent benefit in survival.[5] Overall survival in the entire cohort was 21% at 5 years. Survival in this study was influenced by age greater than 65, depth of chest wall invasion, completeness of resection, and nodal involvement. A larger retrospective study that combined the experience of 3 centers in France (N = 309 patients treated with en bloc resection) showed no benefit to adjuvant radiation in T3N0 patients who underwent en bloc resection.[14] In contrast, adjuvant radiation in patients with resected T3N1 or T3N2 (stage IIIA) disease did experience increased survival.

ROLE OF MULTIMODALITY THERAPY

Excluding lung cancers that invade the apical chest wall or thoracic inlet, studies evaluating multimodality therapy for lung cancers invading other parts of the chest wall are few. Overall survival for T3N0 nonsmall cell lung cancer is 41% in the seventh edition TNM staging, which is inferior to results from multimodality therapy for superior sulcus tumors. If a surgeon can achieve a complete en bloc resection, why employ more modalities for cure? Some have put forth the argument that induction therapy may increase the rate of resectability, influence a complete pathologic response (which has been associated with improved survival), and control micrometastases. Kawaguchi and colleagues studied lung cancer invading the chest wall prospectively in 51 patients with T3N0, T3N1 who received 2 cycles of chemotherapy (cisplatin/venorelbine) concurrently with 40 Gy radiation followed by resection.[22] Some superior sulcus tumors were included in this multi-institutional study, and PET staging was not mandatory. Recurrence was observed in 25% of the patients, where locoregional recurrence was 10%. The median follow-up was only 16 months, with a 2-year overall survival of 85%. Complete pathologic response was identified in only 25% of patients, perhaps due to the lower radiation dose.

The 2016 National Comprehensive Care Network guideline for nonsmall cell lung cancer involving the chest wall recommends surgery as the primary treatment modality for patients with T3N0-1 or T4N0-1 disease, reserving adjuvant chemotherapy with or without radiation for incomplete (R1 or R2) resection.[23] Preoperative chemotherapy or concurrent chemoradiotherapy can also be considered in carefully selected patients with similar disease that is amenable to complete resection. Definitive concurrent chemoradiotherapy is recommended

Table 1
Outcomes of larger retrospective studies since 1999 in Non-Small Cell Lung Cancer patients treated with en bloc chest wall resection

Study	N	Mortality (%)	5-y Survival (%)	Local Recurrence (%)	Distant Recurrence (%)
Downey et al,[11] 1999[a]	334	6	32	19	50
Chapelier et al,[25] 2000	100	4	18	13	45
Magdeleinat et al,[5] 2001	201	7	21	10	8
Facciolo et al,[18] 2001	104	0	61	3	22
Doddoli et al,[14] 2005	309	8	31	57	NR
Deslauriers et al,[27] 2013	125	6	31	43	50

Abbreviation: NR, not reported.
  [a] The survival and recurrence is reported for R0 resection (N = 175).

in patients with lung cancer invading the chest wall with pathologically proven N2 disease.

PROGNOSTIC FACTORS

Review of survival and recurrence in large retrospective series (**Table 1**) evaluating en bloc resection of chest wall invasive non-small cell lung reveals a 32% average 5-year overall survival with a high rate of locoregional and systemic recurrence. Factors that predict poor outcome in this patient population have not really changed over the past 30 years. Incomplete resection remains the most reproducible independent predictor of poor survival in all published series. The absence of lymph node metastases (T3N0 disease) consistently has superior outcome across published series, reaching as high as approximately 70% 5-year survival.[18] The presence of N1 or N2 disease portends worse survival in several published series reporting on the surgical management of chest wall invasion of lung cancer.[3,14,24,25] The Memorial Sloan-Kettering Group reported 49% 5-year survival in completely resected T3N0 disease compared with 27% in T3N1 disease and 15% in T3N2 disease ($P<.0003$).[11] Some studies showed no survival advantage between N1 versus N2 disease.[5,26] The depth of chest wall invasion into parietal pleura has not consistently been associated with worse outcome. Lastly, 2 studies[14,25] reported that the extent of chest wall resection (assessed by the number of ribs removed and not the tumor-free margin) was a predictor of survival. This prognostic factor is likely a surrogate for tumor size.

SUMMARY

Although surgical techniques and approaches to lung cancer invading the chest wall have

incrementally evolved over the past decades, a curative strategy for this disease is predicated on the ability to achieve a complete en bloc resection in the face of limited to no lymph node involvement. N2 disease remains a relative contraindication to surgical resection, except in carefully selected patients with exceptional performance status, where expected outcomes will not exceed 15% to 21% 5-year survival. Despite evidence that supports induction chemoradiotherapy for superior sulcus tumors, there is little evidence to support chemotherapy or radiation around completely resected T3N0 disease. Although many studies suggest that T3N1 disease has worse outcome compared with N0 disease, most surgeons will offer en bloc resection of chest wall and lung since the hilar (N1) disease can be encompassed in a complete resection. Chemotherapy should strongly be considered in this patient population, but timing of delivery (preoperative vs postoperative) remains undetermined. Surgeons need to be well versed in the technical aspects of these operations, including understanding the merits and limitations of all available reconstructive strategies.

REFERENCES

1. Goldstraw P, Crowley J, Chansky K, et al. The IASLC Lung Cancer Staging Project: proposals for the revision of the TNM stage groupings in the forthcoming (seventh) edition of the TNM Classification of malignant tumours. J Thorac Oncol 2007;2(8):706–14.

2. Goldstraw P, Chansky K, Crowley J, et al. The iaslc lung cancer staging project: proposals for revision of the TNM stage groupings in the forthcoming (Eighth) edition of the TNM classification for lung cancer. J Thorac Oncol 2016;11(1):39–51.

3. Piehler JM, Pairolero PC, Weiland LH, et al. Bronchogenic carcinoma with chest wall invasion: factors

affecting survival following en bloc resection. Ann Thorac Surg 1982;34(6):684–91.

4. McCaughan BC, Martini N, Bains MS, et al. Chest wall invasion in carcinoma of the lung. Therapeutic and prognostic implications. J Thorac Cardiovasc Surg 1985;89(6):836–41.

5. Magdeleinat P, Alifano M, Benbrahem C, et al. Surgical treatment of lung cancer invading the chest wall: results and prognostic factors. Ann Thorac Surg 2001;71(4):1094–9.

6. Shaw RR, Paulson DL, Kee JL. Treatment of superior sulcus tumor by irradiation followed by resection. Ann Surg 1961;154(1):29–40.

7. Wright CD, Moncure AC, Shepard JA, et al. Superior sulcus lung tumors. Results of combined treatment (irradiation and radical resection). J Thorac Cardiovasc Surg 1987;94(1):69–74.

8. Attar S, Krasna MJ, Sonett JR, et al. Superior sulcus (Pancoast) tumor: experience with 105 patients. Ann Thorac Surg 1998;66(1):193–8.

9. Rusch VW, Parekh KR, Leon L, et al. Factors determining outcome after surgical resection of T3 and T4 lung cancers of the superior sulcus. J Thorac Cardiovasc Surg 2000;119(6):1147–53.

10. Coleman FP. Primary carcinoma of the lung, with invasion of the ribs: pneumonectomy and simultaneous block resection of the chest wall. Ann Surg 1947;126(2):156–68.

11. Downey RJ, Martini N, Rusch VW, et al. Extent of chest wall invasion and survival in patients with lung cancer. Ann Thorac Surg 1999;68(1):188–93.

12. Ginsberg RJ, Martini N, Zaman M, et al. Influence of surgical resection and brachytherapy in the management of superior sulcus tumor. Ann Thorac Surg 1994;57(6):1440–5.

13. Attar S, Miller JE, Satterfield J, et al. Pancoast's tumor: irradiation or surgery? Ann Thorac Surg 1979; 28(6):578–86.

14. Doddoli C, D'Journo B, Le Pimpec-Barthes F, et al. Lung cancer invading the chest wall: a plea for en-bloc resection but the need for new treatment strategies. Ann Thorac Surg 2005;80(6):2032–40.

15. Dartevelle PG, Chapelier AR, Macchiarini P, et al. Anterior transcervical-thoracic approach for radical resection of lung tumors invading the thoracic inlet. J Thorac Cardiovasc Surg 1993;105(6):1025–34.

16. Rusch VW, Giroux DJ, Kraut MJ, et al. Induction chemoradiation and surgical resection for superior sulcus non-small-cell lung carcinomas: long-term results of Southwest Oncology Group Trial 9416 (Intergroup Trial 0160). J Clin Oncol 2007;25(3):313–8.

17. Kunitoh H, Kato H, Tsuboi M, et al. Phase II trial of preoperative chemoradiotherapy followed by surgical resection in patients with superior sulcus non-small-cell lung cancers: report of Japan Clinical Oncology Group trial 9806. J Clin Oncol 2008; 26(4):644–9.

18. Facciolo F, Cardillo G, Lopergolo M, et al. Chest wall invasion in non-small cell lung carcinoma: a rationale for en bloc resection. J Thorac Cardiovasc Surg 2001;121(4):649–56.

19. Akata S, Kajiwara N, Park J, et al. Evaluation of chest wall invasion by lung cancer using respiratory dynamic MRI. J Med Imaging Radiat Oncol 2008; 52(1):36–9.

20. Albertucci M, DeMeester TR, Rothberg M, et al. Surgery and the management of peripheral lung tumors adherent to the parietal pleura. J Thorac Cardiovasc Surg 1992;103(1):8–12 [discussion: 12–3].

21. Patterson GA, Ilves R, Ginsberg RJ, et al. The value of adjuvant radiotherapy in pulmonary and chest wall resection for bronchogenic carcinoma. Ann Thorac Surg 1982;34(6):692–7.

22. Kawaguchi K, Yokoi K, Niwa H, et al. Trimodality therapy for lung cancer with chest wall invasion: initial results of a phase II study. Ann Thorac Surg 2014;98(4):1184–91.

23. Ettinger DS, Wood DE, Akerley W, et al. NCCN guidelines insights: non-small cell lung cancer, version 4.2016. J Natl Compr Canc Netw 2016; 14(3):255–64.

24. Voltolini L, Rapicetta C, Luzzi L, et al. Lung cancer with chest wall involvement: predictive factors of long-term survival after surgical resection. Lung Cancer 2006;52(3):359–64.

25. Chapelier A, Fadel E, Macchiarini P, et al. Factors affecting long-term survival after en-bloc resection of lung cancer invading the chest wall. Eur J Cardiothorac Surg 2000;18(5):513–8.

26. Casillas M, Paris F, Tarrazona V, et al. Surgical treatment of lung carcinoma involving the chest wall. Eur J Cardiothorac Surg 1989;3(5):425–9.

27. Deslauriers J, Tronc F, Fortin D. Management of tumors involving the chest wall including pancoast tumors and tumors invading the spine. Thorac Surg Clin 2013;23(3):313–25.

Prosthetic Reconstruction of the Chest Wall

Onkar V. Khullar, MD, Felix G. Fernandez, MD, MSc*

KEYWORDS

• Chest wall • Biologic mesh • Prosthetic mesh • Methylmethacrylate • Osteosynthesis

KEY POINTS

- Less than one-third of patients undergoing chest wall resection will require prosthetic reconstruction.
- Prosthetic reconstruction should be limited to resections larger than 5 cm, including 4 or more ribs, including the sternum, and/or located on the lateral or infero-anterior chest wall.
- A variety of materials are available for reconstruction, including synthetic and biological meshes, flexible and rigid patches, and metal osteosynthesis systems.
- The prosthesis should be carefully sized and implanted in order to create a tight closure to avoid billowing and paradoxic motion with respiration.
- Prosthetic chest wall reconstruction can be completed with excellent functional and cosmetic results.

INTRODUCTION

Resection of the chest wall is at times necessary for several conditions, including neoplasms, congenital defects, radiation injuries, and complicated infections. Such resections often result in large defects of the chest wall, which can lead to skeletal instability, altered respiratory mechanics, and significant cosmetic defects. Reconstruction of these large defects of the chest wall can present an arduous challenge for even the most experienced surgeons.

Overall, there are 6 objectives to reconstruction of the chest wall (**Box 1**). The surgical approach to chest wall reconstruction can be divided into 2 phases completed in single stage surgery:

- Restoration of skeletal integrity
- Soft tissue coverage/reconstruction

Here, the authors review the indications, alloplastic materials available (synthetic, biological, and metallic), and surgical technique for prosthetic reconstruction of the skeletal chest wall. Further discussion of autologous flap reconstruction, however, is completed elsewhere in this issue.

INDICATIONS FOR RECONSTRUCTION

Thoughtful consideration should be given when determining which patients require skeletal reconstruction. Careful consideration regarding chest wall stability and integrity is of paramount importance as, in the case of large defects, this may have a substantial impact on postoperative respiratory mechanics and quality of life.[1–3] In fact, most patients who undergo limited resections will not require any prosthetic reconstruction for stabilization. Typically, resections involving 2 to 3 ribs, or less, do not require stabilization of the chest wall. Soft tissue reconstruction alone is all that is needed in these situations. However, larger defects (>5 cm) including 4 or more ribs will typically require skeletal reconstruction with either biological, alloplastic, or synthetic materials.[4] Location of the defect must also be carefully considered. Defects located under the scapula posteriorly or the pectoralis major muscle anteriorly typically do not require prostheses as these structures provide sufficient coverage and rigidity. Similarly, posterior chest wall resections adjacent to the spine typically do not require reconstruction for

Section of General Thoracic Surgery, Emory University School of Medicine, 1365 Clifton Road, NE, Suite A2214, Atlanta, GA 30322, USA
* Corresponding author.
E-mail address: felix.fernandez@emoryhealthcare.org

Thorac Surg Clin 27 (2017) 201–208
http://dx.doi.org/10.1016/j.thorsurg.2017.01.014

Box 1
Objectives of chest wall resection

- Restoration of chest wall rigidity
- Prevention of lung herniation
- Avoiding contraction of the chest wall
- Prevention of trapping of the scapula, particularly when resection involves ribs 5 and 6
- Protect underlying mediastinal organs after sternal resection
- Good cosmetic result

stability. On the other hand, lateral or infero-anterior resections, along with resections of the sternum, will typically require prosthetic reconstruction both for stability as well as coverage of vital intrathoracic structures given the relative lack of major muscle coverage in these areas.

The impact of chest wall resection on pulmonary function remains somewhat controversial. The available literature on this topic is limited to mostly retrospective data, clouded by varying degrees of pulmonary resection required and limitations from selection bias. Certainly, smaller resections will have little effect on pulmonary function. Traditional teaching suggests that larger resections can result in flail segments and paradoxic respiration. There is little available literature to support or refute this teaching, though it does make some degree of physiologic sense. Rigid stabilization of the chest wall in this setting may result in decreased postoperative ventilator requirement, improved pulmonary function, and less discomfort.[5–7] In fact, one study examining long-term results of full-thickness chest wall resection did not identify a difference in preoperative and postoperative pulmonary function after chest wall resection with prosthetic reconstruction and a potentially greater reduction in postoperative pulmonary function if no prosthesis was used.[1]

PROSTHETIC MATERIALS AVAILABLE

The first reported use of a metal prosthesis was in 1909.[8] With significant advances and refinement, a variety of materials are now available to the surgeon for prosthetic chest wall reconstruction, including biologic, alloplastic, and synthetic materials (**Box 2**). The ideal prosthetic material for chest wall reconstruction should have the following characteristics.

- Rigid enough to abolish paradoxic chest wall motion
- Malleable enough to allow for appropriate contouring
- Physically and chemically inert

Box 2
Materials used for chest wall reconstruction/ stabilization

Synthetic mesh
- Methylmethacrylate
- Polyglactin (Vicryl, Ethicon, Inc, Somerville, NJ)
- Nylon
- Polypropylene (Marlex, Davol & Bard, Cranston, RI, and Prolene, Ethicon Inc, Somerville, NJ)
- Polytetrafluoroethylene (Dualmesh, W.L. Gore & Associates, Flagstaff, AZ)
- Silastic
- Silicone

Bioprosthetic materials
- AlloDerm (LifeCell Corporation, Branchburg, NJ)
  - Cadaveric human dermis
- Surgisis (Cook Biomedical, Bloomington, IN)
  - Porcine small intestine submucosa
- Permacol (Covidien, Norwalk, CT)
  - Porcine dermis
- XenMtrix (Davol Inc, Warwick, RI)
  - Porcine dermis
- Strattice (LifeCell Corporation, Branchburg, NJ)
  - Porcine dermis
- Tutopatch (RTI Surgical, Alachua, FL)
  - Bovine pericardium
- Veritas (Baxter, Deerfield, IL)
  - Bovine pericardium
- SurgiMend (Integra Life Sciences, Plainsboro, NJ)
  - Bovine dermis

Osteosynthesis systems
- Stratos (MedXpert GmbH, Heitersheim, Germany)
  - Titanium
- MatrixRIB Fixation (DePuy Synthes, West Chester, PA)
  - Titanium
- Stainless steel bars

- Allows for tissue in-growth
- Radiolucent
- Sterile and resistant to infection
- Inexpensive

Unfortunately, no such ideal material is available. Typically, a combination of these materials, with or without myocutaneous flaps, is required for complex composite reconstructions. Often, choice of material is dictated by surgeon or institution preference and anecdotal experience given a paucity of literature comparing one material to another.

Synthetic Meshes and Patches

There are a variety of synthetic materials at the surgeon's disposal for chest wall reconstruction. Both rigid (methylmethacrylate) and flexible (various meshes) are available (see **Box 2**). Although each material has advantages and disadvantages, there are little data available comparing these materials. As a result, the choice of material used is often based on institutional availability and surgeon preference. Flexible meshes, such as vicryl and polypropylene, have several major advantages in the use of chest wall reconstruction. They are easily manipulated and can be stretched in all directions in order to create a taut closure with uniformly distributed tension, thereby avoiding paradoxic motion. Additionally, they can prevent the formation of a seroma as they are permeable to body fluids.

However, the same permeability can make it difficult to control the pleural space and effusions. The authors' preference is to use a flexible patch for reconstruction when rigidity is not required, most often with a nonabsorbable synthetic polytetrafluoroethylene (PTFE) patch. They are similarly easily manipulated and stretched (**Fig. 1**A) and can be used to create a watertight closure (**Fig. 1**B). As a result, they can function as an excellent scaffold for a myocutaneous flap, if needed. If implanted correctly, there should be no postoperative paradoxic chest wall motion with respiration. There are several disadvantages

of such patches, however, that must be noted. If not kept tight when sewing, they can billow into the chest with breathing, as they are not rigid. Additionally, they can loosen over time. More importantly, as they are impermeable, they must be removed if they become infected.

Occasionally, when reconstructing very large defects, such as those from resection of several ribs or resection of the manubrium and sternum, a more rigid patch is required. Most commonly, methylmethacrylate is used, sandwiched between 2 layers of mesh, typically made of polypropylene (Marlex, Bard Davol, Warwick, RI). Such a prosthesis is prepared and shaped on the back table and can, therefore, be customized to each individual patient and chest wall defect (**Fig. 2**). The polymer is shaped such that a sewing ring of mesh extends several centimeters beyond the hardened methylmethacrylate.[9] This ring is then secured to the surrounding skeletal structure as discussed later (see **Fig. 2**A). Lardinois and colleagues[2] have described a modification to this technique that lowers the viscosity of the methylmethacrylate, thereby slowing the time required for hardening. Thus, the sandwich may be modeled in situ, allowing for easier customization of the patch.

Such a rigid chest wall reconstruction has several advantages and disadvantages. It provides excellent chest wall stability, which may theoretically result in less respiratory complications. Additionally, given its rigidity, it can provide superior coverage of vital mediastinal structures when used to reconstruct the sternum (see **Fig. 2**A, B). Finally, it is relatively inexpensive when compared with other materials used for reconstruction. Unfortunately, methylmethacrylate prostheses have been associated with higher rates of wound complications, such as seromas, hematomas, and infections, requiring removal in up to 5% of patients.[7]

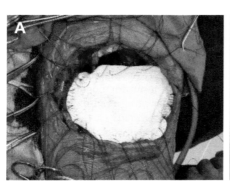 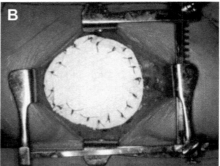

Fig. 1. A nonabsorbable synthetic PTFE patch (Dualmesh, W.L. Gore & Associates, Flagstaff, AZ) is used to reconstruct the lateral chest wall. Synthetic patches are easily manipulated and stretched (*A*) and can be used to create a watertight closure (*B*).

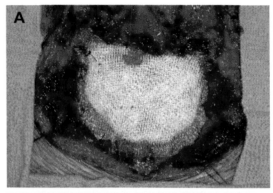

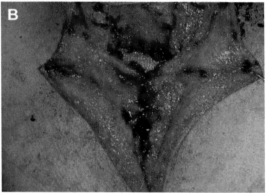

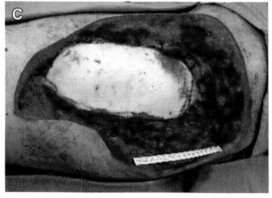

Fig. 2. Chest wall reconstruction with a composite sandwich prosthesis, made of methylmethacrylate encased in polypropylene (Marlex) mesh. (*A*) The prosthesis is used to reconstruct the manubrium after resection, providing rigid coverage of the mediastinum and skeletal stability. (*B*) Soft tissue flaps are used to cover the prosthesis. (*C*) Methylmethacrylate can also be used for rigid reconstruction of large, lateral chest wall defects.

Biological Mesh

The number of bioprosthetic meshes available has increased considerably in the last 20 years, and it has gained in popularity (see **Box 2**). These meshes function as decellularized biological scaffold allowing for potentially greater tissue ingrowth while maintaining structural integrity. They are gradually revascularized and remodeled into autologous tissue. Finally, and perhaps most importantly, they may be more resistant to infection.[10] As a result, they are often used for reconstruction in infected fields. Unfortunately, there are only a few studies examining the use of bioprosthetic materials in chest wall reconstruction.[11] The technique for implantation is similar to other meshes as described earlier. Maintaining appropriate physiologic tension when using biological meshes is particularly important. As tissue ingrowth and remodeling occurs, material laxity can ensue leading to bulging. As a result, they are often used in combination with the myocutaneous flap coverage. For these reasons, combined with relatively higher costs, these materials are infrequently used.

Osteosynthesis Systems

Osteosynthesis systems are metallic-based systems used for bridging multiple rib and/or sternal defects (**Fig. 3**). These systems can provide a creative method for reconstructing the rigid support structure of the chest wall and may allow for more physiologic rib movement than what can be achieved with methylmethacrylate or other mesh prostheses. However, they still typically need to be used in combination with one of the aforementioned meshes and/or a myocutaneous flap to cover complex chest wall defects and for control of the pleural space.[12]

The two most common osteosynthesis systems are the titanium-based Stratos (MedXpert GmbH, Heitersheim, Germany) and the MatrixRIB Fixation (DePuy Synthes, West Chester, PA) systems. Implantation techniques for these are specific to the system being used. For example, utilization of the Stratos system entails crimping titanium clips onto the rib or sternal edges, followed by a bridging titanium bar. The MatrixRIB system is screwed directly into the bony edges on both sides of the defect.

Given their higher tensile strength and potentially greater resistance to infection, titanium implant systems for chest wall rigid fixation are favored over other rigid metals, such as stainless steel and ceramic. However, one retrospective study did note failure of the titanium implant in 44% of patients due to either broken or displaced implants.[13] Additionally, osteosynthesis systems will have less tissue ingrowth than most meshes and may, therefore, be subject to higher rates of infection, which would necessitate removal of the implants.

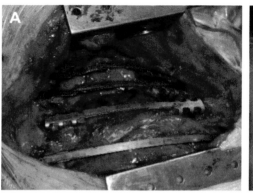 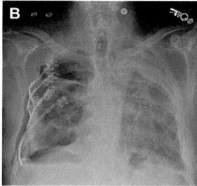

Fig. 3. (*A*) A titanium osteosynthesis system used to bridge multiple rib defects after lateral chest wall resection. (*B*) Postoperative chest radiograph.

SURGICAL TECHNIQUE

Regardless of material chosen, there are several principles that must be adhered to when implanting a mesh prosthesis. The surgeon should always remember that the goal of prosthetic chest wall reconstruction is to create a rigid surface in order to avoid paradoxic motion, lung herniation, and so forth. Therefore, the mesh should be contoured to the defect and tailored to allow for enough room for adequate suturing. The interrupted horizontal mattress suture of a permanent synthetic material is the suture of choice. Although a simple running suture may be more expeditious, interrupted sutures allow for the small adjustments needed to keep the prosthesis taught.

Typically, the mesh is secured around a rib at the firmest point of the resection margin. If the surgeon is not able to secure the prosthesis around the around the rib, sutures should be placed through the rib periosteum. Sutures are then placed radially around the defect, progressively tightening the prosthesis until it is secured circumferentially (see **Fig. 1**A). For irregularly shaped defects, composite prostheses often using multiple pieces of either the same or different prosthesis are required (see **Fig. 2**). Accordingly, the surgeon must be both flexible and creative in customizing the reconstruction to each individual patient.

CLINICAL OUTCOMES

A review of the literature regarding clinical outcomes after chest wall resection and prosthetic reconstruction is limited by a lack of quality prospective research. The existing literature is composed of a few retrospective case series that look only at synthetic meshes and patches (**Table 1**). Even fewer studies compare the numerous prostheses head-to-head. Finally, there are no significant studies examining biological meshes and only a few small case reports and series for osteosyntheses systems in chest wall reconstruction.[12–15] As a result, current practice is directed by these few limited case series and anecdotal surgeon experience.

In the largest series to date and the only one to compare 2 techniques head-to-head, Weyant and colleagues[7] reported a series of 262 patients who underwent chest wall resection, comparing reconstruction with a rigid prosthesis (Marlex methylmethacrylate sandwich, n = 112), nonrigid prosthesis (polypropylene or PTFE mesh, n = 97), and no prosthesis (n = 53). They found no difference in overall complication rates between the 3 techniques. However, methylmethacrylate was associated with slightly higher rates of wound complications, such as seromas, hematomas, and infections, when compared with a patch (8.0% vs 3.1%, P = .05). The rate of prosthesis removal was 4.3% overall and was not significantly different between the two prostheses. In fact, rates of synthetic prosthesis removal (typically related to infectious complications) ranged from only 2.5% to 8.0% across the various studies (see **Table 1**). The exact incidence of mesh infections is unclear, though should be uncommon. Similarly, there are no published studies to date examining the use of antibiotics to prevent prosthetic mesh infection when used for chest wall reconstruction. The literature in regard to antibiotic use in abdominal wall hernias still remains somewhat controversial as well. The authors' routine practice is to give a perioperative dose of a second-generation cephalosporin within 1 hour of incision, periodically redosed during the operation, followed by 2 postoperative doses. This practice provides 24 hours total of perioperative antibiotic prophylaxis.

Table 1
Select previously published series of prosthetic chest wall reconstruction with synthetic mesh

Author	No. With Prosthetic Reconstruction	Mesh Used	Overall Complications (%)	Prosthesis Removal (%)	Mortality (%)
Deschamps et al,[16] 1999	197	Polypropylene and PTFE mesh	46.2	2.5[a]	4.1
Lardinois et al,[2] 2000	26	Methylmethacrylate	23.0	7.7	0
Mansour et al,[17] 2002	93	Various	24.0	NR	7.0
Weyant et al,[7] 2006	209	Polypropylene-methylmethacrylate sandwich or polypropylene mesh	33.0	4.3	3.8
Daigeler et al,[3] 2009	62	Polypropylene mesh	42.0	6.5	5.4

Abbreviation: NR, not reported.

[a] All in patients (n = 5) who received polypropylene mesh. Four patients with PTFE developed infections but did not require prosthesis removal.

Perhaps the most anticipated complication with use of a foreign material for reconstruction would be wound complications and prosthesis infections. However, these were much less common than other complications. As summarized in **Table 1**, overall complication rates ranged from 23% to 46%.[2,16] Mortality after chest wall resection with reconstruction remained relatively low, ranging from 0% to 7%.[2,17,18] In general, most postoperative complications were respiratory in nature. For example, in a series published by Mansour and colleagues,[17] the two most common complications were pneumonia (14% of patients) and ARDS (6%). Similarly, in one series of 197 patients who underwent prosthetic chest wall reconstruction with either polypropylene or PTFE, 24.4% of patients suffered a respiratory-related complication, representing more than half of the complications in the study.[16]

Although this overall complication rate is relatively high, it does not seem to be related to the use of a prosthesis and seems to be more a function of chest wall resection. Several of these series retrospectively compared the use of a prosthesis with no prosthesis and found no correlation with postoperative complication occurrence.[1,3,7,18] For instance, Weyant and colleagues,[7] in a multivariable analysis of predictors of complications after chest wall resection, found no correlation between complications and the use of a nonrigid or rigid prosthesis. Moreover, the only significant predictors for postoperative complications were age, lobectomy/pneumonectomy, and the size of chest wall defect.

The available literature regarding outcomes with titanium osteosyntheses systems is limited to several small case series. One series of 31 patients reconstructed with titanium implants and PTFE mesh showed encouraging results, with successful reconstruction in most patients, only 2 cases of wound infection that required implant removal in 1 patient, and only a single respiratory complication, potentially due to greater chest wall rigidity.[12] However, a follow-up study from the same investigators reported an implant failure rate of 44%, due to either broken or displaced implants. Interestingly, the mean duration to implant failure was 6.6 months. The greatest risk for implant failure was use of the titanium bars in an anterior chest wall location. This finding led the investigators to conclude that if used in this location, consideration should be given to early removal of the titanium implants.[13]

Aside from occurrence of postoperative complications, the other important clinical result to consider when evaluating chest wall reconstruction is long-term functional outcomes.

Few studies have evaluated long-term pulmonary function and patient-reported quality-of-life results.[1–3] There is a theoretic benefit of chest wall stabilization in order to avoid paradoxic chest wall motion, thereby maintaining pulmonary function. However, this has not been definitively shown in the limited existing literature as no studies have clearly shown diminished pulmonary function without the use of a prosthesis. This determination is further clouded by the limitations of retrospective data and selection bias, in that patients with limited pulmonary function would be less likely to undergo extensive chest wall resections and/or reconstruction.

Lardinois and colleagues[2] published a series of 26 patients undergoing reconstruction with methylmethacrylate and found that pulmonary function was maintained 6 months after reconstruction, with no difference in forced expiratory volume in 1 second (FEV_1) when compared with preoperative values. In a larger, more recent series, FEV_1 in patients reconstructed with a synthetic prosthesis was reduced by only 4.1% postoperatively, compared with 17.5% when no prosthesis was used in the same series; however, this difference was not statistically significant.[1] In another series, the use of a nonrigid prosthesis was associated with lower rates of ventilator support when compared with autologous tissue reconstruction only (33% vs 60%), though again this result did not reach statistical significance ($P = .19$).[19] Therefore, based on the available literature, we can likely conclude that prosthetic chest wall reconstruction is able to maintain preoperative pulmonary function. Further study is needed to determine whether there is a significant advantage to prosthetic reconstruction over reconstruction without prosthesis.

However, what does seem to be clear is the lasting effects of chest wall reconstruction on quality of life. In a series of 92 consecutive patients undergoing chest wall resection, 62 of whom received a Prolene (Ethicon, Inc, Somerville, NJ) mesh implant, quality-of-life parameters in long-term survivors were significantly reduced in regard to activity levels and manageable volume of work several years after surgery. Most long-term survivors also had some degree of sensation disorders or motion-related pain. Further, nearly 70% of patients who presented for long-term follow-up showed paradoxic chest wall movement of at least 0.5 cm, with no correlation to the use of a prosthetic mesh. Yet, despite these findings, the investigators found that most patients (94%) would undergo the procedure again.[3]

SUMMARY

Although most chest wall resections do not result in a large soft tissue defect and do not require any form of prosthetic reconstruction, approximately one-third of resections will require a prosthesis to close a larger defect. Large chest wall resections can result in skeletal instability, altered respiratory mechanics, and significant cosmetic defects. Prosthetic reconstruction should be limited to resections larger than 5 cm, including 4 or more ribs, including the sternum, and/or located on the lateral or infero-anterior chest wall.

A variety of materials are available for reconstruction, including synthetic and biological meshes, flexible and rigid patches, and metal osteosynthesis systems. The material chosen should be optimized to each patient and defect being reconstructed.

Careful sizing and implantation can result in tight closure, thereby minimizing billowing and paradoxic motion with respiration, often with minimal effect on pulmonary function. If implanted carefully, these defects can be reconstructed with minimal complications and low rates of prosthesis removal. As a result, prosthetic chest wall reconstructions can be safely completed with excellent functional and cosmetic results.

REFERENCES

1. Leuzzi G, Nachira D, Cesario A, et al. Chest wall tumors and prosthetic reconstruction: a comparative analysis on functional outcome. Thorac Cancer 2015;6(3):247–54.

2. Lardinois D, Muller M, Furrer M, et al. Functional assessment of chest wall integrity after methylmethacrylate reconstruction. Ann Thorac Surg 2000; 69(3):919–23.

3. Daigeler A, Druecke D, Hakimi M, et al. Reconstruction of the thoracic wall-long-term follow-up including pulmonary function tests. Langenbecks Arch Surg 2009;394(4):705–15.

4. Ferraro P, Cugno S, Liberman M, et al. Principles of chest wall resection and reconstruction. Thorac Surg Clin 2010;20(4):465–73.

5. Kroll SS, Walsh G, Ryan B, et al. Risks and benefits of using Marlex mesh in chest wall reconstruction. Ann Plast Surg 1993;31(4):303–6.

6. Tanaka H, Yukioka T, Yamaguti Y, et al. Surgical stabilization of internal pneumatic stabilization? A prospective randomized study of management of severe flail chest patients. J Trauma 2002;52(4): 727–32 [discussion: 732].

7. Weyant MJ, Bains MS, Venkatraman E, et al. Results of chest wall resection and reconstruction with and without rigid prosthesis. Ann Thorac Surg 2006; 81(1):279–85.

8. Gangolphe L. Enorme enchondrome de la fourchette sternale. Lyon Chir 1909;2:112.

9. McCormack P, Bains MS, Beattie EJ Jr, et al. New trends in skeletal reconstruction after resection of chest wall tumors. Ann Thorac Surg 1981;31(1): 45–52.

10. Diaz JJ Jr, Conquest AM, Ferzoco SJ, et al. Multi-institutional experience using human acellular dermal matrix for ventral hernia repair in a compromised surgical field. Arch Surg 2009;144(3):209–15.

11. Butler CE, Langstein HN, Kronowitz SJ. Pelvic, abdominal, and chest wall reconstruction with Allo-Derm in patients at increased risk for mesh-related complications. Plast Reconstr Surg 2005;116(5): 1263–75 [discussion: 1276–7].

12. Berthet JP, Wihlm JM, Canaud L, et al. The combination of polytetrafluoroethylene mesh and titanium rib implants: an innovative process for reconstructing large full thickness chest wall defects. Eur J Cardiothorac Surg 2012;42(3):444–53.

13. Berthet JP, Gomez Caro A, Solovei L, et al. Titanium implant failure after chest wall osteosynthesis. Ann Thorac Surg 2015;99(6):1945–52.

14. Fabre D, El Batti S, Singhal S, et al. A paradigm shift for sternal reconstruction using a novel titanium rib bridge system following oncological resections. Eur J Cardiothorac Surg 2012;42(6):965–70.

15. Coonar AS, Wihlm JM, Wells FC, et al. Intermediate outcome and dynamic computerised tomography after chest wall reconstruction with the STRATOS titanium rib bridge system: video demonstration of preserved bucket-handle rib motion. Interact Cardiovasc Thorac Surg 2011;12(1):80–1.

16. Deschamps C, Tirnaksiz BM, Darbandi R, et al. Early and long-term results of prosthetic chest wall reconstruction. J Thorac Cardiovasc Surg 1999;117(3): 588–91 [discussion: 591–2].

17. Mansour KA, Thourani VH, Losken A, et al. Chest wall resections and reconstruction: a 25-year experience. Ann Thorac Surg 2002;73(6):1720–5 [discussion: 1725–6].

18. Losken A, Thourani VH, Carlson GW, et al. A reconstructive algorithm for plastic surgery following extensive chest wall resection. Br J Plast Surg 2004;57(4):295–302.

19. Hanna WC, Ferri LE, McKendy KM, et al. Reconstruction after major chest wall resection: can rigid fixation be avoided? Surgery 2011;150(4):590–7.

Index

Note: Page numbers of article titles are in **boldface** type.

A

Abramson technique
  clinical results of, 130
  modifications to, 130
  patient selection for, 129
  for pectus carinatum, 129, 130
  and postoperative care, 130
  preparation for, 129
  surgical approach for, 129, 130
Actinomyces
  and chest wall infections, 93, 94
Acute chest wall infections: Surgical site infections, necrotizing soft tissue infections, and sternoclavicular joint infection, **73–86**
Adjuvant therapy
  for lung cancer invading chest wall, 197
  for radiation-induced sarcoma, 177, 178
Aneurysmal bone cyst
  and osseous chest wall tumors, 185, 186
Aspergillus
  and chest wall infections, 94

B

Biological mesh
  and chest wall prosthetic reconstruction, 204
Bone tumors
  of the chest wall, 181–191
Breast cancer
  and chest wall irradiation, 171–173, 175–178
Breast cancer invading chest wall
  clinical outcomes of surgery for, 161–162
  complications of surgery for, 162, 163
  and reconstruction, 159, 161–163
  surgery for, 160, 161
Bronchial stump
  vacuum dressings on, 79
Brucella
  and chest wall infections, 93

C

Chemotherapy
  for osseous chest wall tumors, 191
  for sarcomas, 144, 145
Chest drains
  and vacuum dressings, 78
Chest wall
  acute infections of, 73–84

and bone tumors, 181–191
breast cancer invasion of, 159–163
chronic infections of, 87–96
lung cancer invasion of, 195–198
primary osseous tumors of, 181–191
primary soft tissue tumors of, 139–145
prosthetic reconstruction of, 201–208
and radiation treatment, 171–178
reconstruction of, 159, 161–163, 165–169
Chest wall actinomycosis
  and soft tissue infections, 93, 94
Chest wall deformities
  and pectus carinatum, 128–130
  and pectus excavatum, 123–128
  and straight back syndrome, 133–137
Chest wall infections
  and *Actinomyces,* 93, 94
  and *Aspergillus,* 94
  and *Brucella,* 93
  of cartilage and bones, 88–93
  and costochondral infections, 88, 89
  and *Echinococcus,* 94
  and granulomas, 93, 94
  and *Leishmania,* 94
  and necrotizing fasciitis, 73, 79, 80
  and necrotizing soft tissue, 79–81
  and negative pressure wound therapy, 77–79
  and osteomyelitis, 89, 90
  and *Phycomyces,* 94
  and *Pseudomonas aeruginosa,* 90
  and soft tissue, 79–81, 93–95
  and *Staphylococcus aureus,* 88, 90
  and sternoclavicular joint, 81–84
  and surgical site, 73–77
  and thoracotomy, 73–75
  and tuberculosis, 88, 89, 93
  and vacuum-assisted closure, 77–79
Chest wall irradiation
  and breast cancer, 171–173, 175–178
  and lung cancer, 175–178
  and osteonecrosis, 172–174
  and radiation-induced sarcoma, 174–178
  resection after, 172
Chest wall prosthetic reconstruction
  and biological mesh, 204
  clinical outcomes of, 205–207
  indications for, 201, 202
  materials for, 202–205
  objectives of, 202

Thorac Surg Clin 27 (2017) 209–213
http://dx.doi.org/10.1016/S1547-4127(17)30023-3
1547-4127/17

Moving?

Make sure your subscription moves with you!

To notify us of your new address, find your **Clinics Account Number** (located on your mailing label above your name), and contact customer service at:

Email: journalscustomerservice-usa@elsevier.com

800-654-2452 (subscribers in the U.S. & Canada)
314-447-8871 (subscribers outside of the U.S. & Canada)

Fax number: 314-447-8029

Elsevier Health Sciences Division
Subscription Customer Service
3251 Riverport Lane
Maryland Heights, MO 63043

*To ensure uninterrupted delivery of your subscription, please notify us at least 4 weeks in advance of move.

ELSEVIER

Printed and bound by CPI Group (UK) Ltd, Croydon, CR0 4YY

13/05/2025

01869712-0001